BrainChip
for
Pathology

USMLE Step 1 Review

BrainChip
for
Pathology

Georgina Garcia
Class of 2002

University of Iowa College of Medicine
Iowa City, Iowa

Blackwell
Publishing

(c) 2002 by Blackwell Science
a Blackwell Publishing company

Blackwell Publishing, Inc., 350 Main Street, Malden, Massachusetts 02148-5018, USA
Blackwell Science Ltd, Osney Mead, Oxford OX2 0EL, UK
Blackwell Science Asia Pty Ltd, 550 Swanston Street, Carlton, Victoria 3053, Australia
Blackwell Verlag GmbH, Kurfürstendamm 57, 10707 Berlin, Germany

02 03 04 05 5 4 3 2 1

ISBN: 0-632-004639-2

Library of Congress Cataloging-in-Publication Data

Garcia, Georgina (Georgina E.)
    BrainChip for pathology / Georgina Garcia.
      p. ; cm.
    ISBN 0-632-04639-2 (pbk.)
 1. Pathology—Outlines, syllabi, etc. 2. Physicians—Licenses—United
States—Examinations—Study guides.
    [DNLM: 1. Pathology—Outlines. QZ 18.2 G216b 2002] I. Title: Brain
chip for pathology. II. Title.
    RB120 .G37 2002
    616.07—dc21
                                    2002006043

A catalogue record for this title is available from the British Library

Acquisitions: Beverly Copland
Development: Julia Casson
Production: Nancy Duffy
Cover design: GraphCom Corporation
Typesetter: TechBooks, in India
Printed and bound by Walsworth Publishing Company in Missouri

For further information on Blackwell Publishing, visit our website:
www.blackwellscience.com

DEDICATION

This book is dedicated to my parents, Carlos and Miriam Garcia. They have given all of themselves and their lives, so that their children can be and do anything their hearts desire. They have provided me with unwavering love and support in every aspect of my life. I would be nothing without them.

Look for these other books in the BrainChip Series!

BrainChip for Microbiology
BrainChip for Biochemistry

TABLE OF CONTENTS

CHAPTER 3: ENDOCRINE SYSTEM

CHAPTER 4: GASTROINTESTINAL

CHAPTER 5: GENITOURINARY

CHAPTER 6: HEMATOLOGY

CHAPTER 7: NEUROLOGY

CHAPTER 8: RENAL

Chapter 9: Respiratory

PREFACE

Pathology is one of the most complex and important subjects in medical school. It is where all of the first years classes on biochemistry, cell biology, physiology, histology, and anatomy intersect to create the diseases that physicians face every day. As students, it is difficult to find resources that combine pertinent pathophysiology, clinically relevant findings, and treatment regimens. In addition, there is normally a separate set of books that emphasize high yield information tested on the Step 1 of the USMLE. Looking up multiple sources can be frustrating and time consuming. The goal of this book, **BrainChip for Pathology,** is to fulfill all of these needs in one small book that will fit in the pocket of a short white coat.

This book was designed to give a basic understanding of pathology in a clear, concise manner. The book is divided into organ-based chapters. Each disease begins with a clinical vignette and then is described in five ways: pathology, clinical findings, clinical vignettes, diagnosis, and treatment. The vignette highlights patient populations, risk factors, common chief complaints, physical exam findings, and diagnostic results characteristic of each disease. These clinical vignettes can be useful in preparation for Step 1 of the USMLE. Following each clinical scenario is a description of the pathophysiology. It succinctly describes the pathways and mechanisms responsible for each disease process. Then, conveniently there is a list of the clinical manifestations of the disease in the patient. This includes concurrent risk factors, populations at risk, genetic inheritance, and associated syndromes or diseases. Listed below it are the recommended diagnostic tools and current treatments used for the disease. Finally, color photographs are included to remind you of key imaging findings, gross pathology, or histology commonly associated with the disease.

How can you use this book?
- Use it in conjunction with a comprehensive medical textbook during the pathology course.
- Pack it along on the internal medicine wards.
- Use it as a quick reference on a patient.
- Review for Step 1 or 2 of the USMLE.

Remember, learning medicine has been likened to trying to drink information ... from a fire hose. Repetition is good.

Multiple texts, references, review books, and lecture notes have been reviewed to make this book as complete and accurate as possible. Useful mnemonics have been added. Pathognomonic pictures or clinical findings have been highlighted. Hopefully, it provides a concise review of pathology in an easy to read (and carry) format.

While much effort has gone into this book, there are bound to be suggestions and comments. I welcome them. My only hope for this book was to create a useful and practical resource for medical students. This book was written for medical students, by one.

Georgina E. Garcia
Class of 2002
University of Iowa College of Medicine

ACKNOWLEDGEMENTS

There are so many people who contributed to the production of this book.

First, I want to thank Beverly Copland, Julia Casson, and Blackwell Publishing for all of their support throughout this project. Thank you Julia, for all of your energy and hard work. This book is the result of everyone at Blackwell Publishing's dedication and effort.

I am indebted to Barry DeYoung, MD and Mary Stone, MD at the University of Iowa Hospitals and Clinics, Department of Pathology. Dr. DeYoung, you provided me with much more than photos to use in this book, you provided me with true encouragement and mentorship. I would also like to thank Dr. Mary Stone for her wonderful contribution of dermatology images.

Finally, I would like to thank the Joe and Jeannie for believing and supporting me when I came up with the crazy idea of writing a book while in medical school. Again, thank you to my family, including my siblings Carlos, Jasmin, and Rebecca—I love you.

—Georgina E. Garcia

Abbreviations

Ab	Antibody
ACE	Angiotensin converting enzyme
ACTH	Adrenocortiocotropic hormone
AFP	Alpha fetoprotein
Ag	Antigen
ALT(SGPT)	Alanine aminotransferase
Anti-DNA	Anti double stranded DNA
AST(SGOT)	Aspartate transferase
BUN	Blood urea nitrogen
CAB	Coronary artery bypass
CBC	Complete blood count
CEA	Carcinoembryonic antigen
CHF	Congestive heart failure
CK-MB	Creatine kinase MB
CMV	Cytomegalovirus
CNS	Central nervous system
CRP	C reactive protein
CSF	Cerebral spinal fluid
CT	Computed tomography
CXR	Chest X-ray
DEXA	Dual energy x-ray absorptiometry
DIP	Distal interphalangeal joint
EBV	Epstein-Barr virus
EKG	Electrocardiogram
ELISA	Enzyme-linked immunosorbent assay
ETOH	Ethanol
EMG	Electromyogram
ERCP	Endoscopic retrograde cholangiopancreatography
ESR	Erythrocyte sedimentation rate
FTA-ABS	Fluorescent treponemal antibody/absorption
GABA	γ-Aminobutyric acid
(G)BM	Glomerular basement membrane
GGT	Gamma-glutamyltranspeptidase
GI	Gastrointestinal
GnRH	Gonadotropin-releasing hormone
HA	Headache
HCG	Human chorionic gonadotropin
HEENT	Head, eyes, ears, neck, and throat exam

HEP	Hepatitis
HIV	Human immunodeficiency virus
HLA	Human leukocyte antigen
HPV	Human papillomavirus
HSV	Herpes simplex virus
HTN	Hypertension
IVIG	Intravenous immunoglobin
JVD	Jugular venous distension
LDH	Lactate dehydrogenase
LP	Lumbar puncture
LV	Left ventricle
MCV	Mean corpuscular volume
MRI	Magnetic resonance imaging
MVA	Motor vehicle accident
NSAID	Nonsteroidal anti-inflammatory drug
P-ANCA	Antineutrophil cytoplasmic autoantibodies
PCTA	Percutaneous transluminal angioplasty
PE	Physical examination
PFT	Pulmonary function test
PIP	Proximal interphalangeal joint
PMN	Polymorphonuclear leukocytes
PSA	Prostate specific antigen
PT	Prothrombin time
PTH	Parathyroid hormone
PTT	Partaial thromboplastin time
PUVA	Psoralen + UVA light
RH	Rhesus factor
RLQ	Right lower quadrant
RPR	Ribonucleoprotein
RSV	Respiratory syncytial virus
SLE	Systemic lupus erythematosis
TB	Tuberculosis
TIA	Transient ischemic attack
TRH	Thyroid releasing hormone
TSH	Thyroid stimulating hormone
UA	Urinary analysis
UGT	Uridine diphosphate-glucuronosyltransferase
URI	Upper respiratory infection
US	Ultrasound
UTI	Urinary tract infection
UVB	Ultraviolet B
VA	Veterans Association
VDRL	Venereal Disease Research Lab
WBC	White blood cells/count

CHAPTER 1
CARDIOLOGY

History of Present Illness: A 54-year-old white male is brought into the emergency department for **chest pain.** He reports that it started early this morning shortly after he woke up. He clutches his right hand over his heart and sternal area when asked where the pain is. He also has some **shortness of breath** and **diaphoreses.** A preliminary EKG on intake shows elevated ST segments in leads III, IV.

Disease: Acute Myocardial Infarction

Pathology: Coronary occlusion **atherosclerotic plaque (most common),** vasospasm, emboli, hematologic abnormalities, vasculitis, aortic dissection, cocaine → **ischemia** → coagulative necrosis (day 1) → acute inflammation, vessel dilation, neutrophil infiltrate (day 2–4) → granulation tissue (day 5–10) → scar tissue (week 7) (Figs. 1.1 and 1.2).

Characteristics: Males > females. **Shortness of breath; nausea;** fatigue; diaphoresis; syncope; hypertension; **chest pain** radiating to the left shoulder, arm, and jaw. Can be **asymptomatic.** Complications include cardiac **arrhythmia,** LV failure, pulmonary edema, cardiogenic

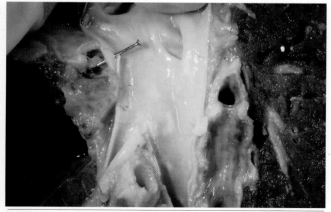

FIGURE 1.1 A therosclerotic plague. © *Barry R. DeYoung, MD, University of Iowa College of Medicine.*

1

CARDIOLOGY—cont'd

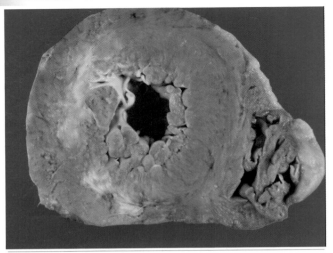

FIGURE 1.2 Acute myocardial infarction. © *Barry R. DeYoung, MD, University of Iowa College of Medicine.*

shock, mitral insufficiency, ventricular aneurysm, cardiac rupture, fibrinous pericarditis.

Diagnosis: Clinical diagnosis; EKG ST elevation or depression and Q waves; Troponin (first 8 hr); CK-MB (24 hr); LDH (2–7 days); AST; echocardiogram showing abnormal wall movement; Technetium-99m pyrophosphate scintigraphy; blood pressure.

Treatment: Thrombolytic; t-PA; streptokinase; anisoylated plasminogen streptokinase activator complex (APSAC); acute PTCA; nitroglycerin; analgesia; beta-blockers; oxygen; aspirin. Long-term beta-blockers; ACE inhibitors; calcium channel blockers; anticoagulation; antiarrhythmics.

History of Present Illness: A 27-year-old male presents with **chest pain.** He says that it is a 5/10 pain that came on yesterday. It gets worse with exertion and is not positional in nature. His past medical history is significant for dispnea and new onset of **syncope** once this past month. On physical exam you note a harsh **crescendo-decrescendo systolic ejection murmur at the left sternal border that radiates to the neck.** It is also noted that he has a diminished carotid pulse.

Disease: Aortic Stenosis

Pathology: (1) Congenital bicuspid valve; (2) Infectious (rheumatic fever); (3) Aortic calcification of normal valves with age-related changes or congenitally bicuspid valves. → ↑ left ventricular pressure → left ventricular hypertrophy → ↑ oxygen demand/ ↓ coronary artery perfusion→ angina and syncope → CHF (Fig. 1.3).

Characteristics: Adults who are asymptomatic until middle or late life. Delayed/diminished carotid pulses; harsh **crescendo-decrescendo systolic ejection** murmur; **angina; syncope;** fatigue; dyspnea; CHF; congenital bicuspid aortic valve; palpable left ventricular thrill; paradoxical splitting of S_2; arrhythmias.

Diagnosis: Clinical diagnosis; EKG left ventricular hypertrophy; x-ray showing calcified valve; echocardiogram illustrating calcification and left ventricular function; cardiac catheterization ↓ valve gradient.

Treatment: Valvuloplasty; valve replacement; anticoagulation; diuretics; prophylactic antibiotics prior to surgical procedures.

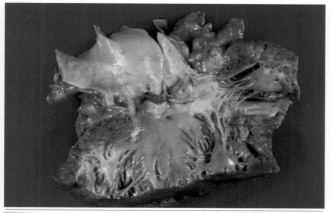

FIGURE 1.3 Aortic stenosis. © *Barry R. DeYoung, MD, University of Iowa College of Medicine.*

History of Present Illness: A 32-year-old male presents with a 3-day history of fever and **hematemesis.** He has been having severe asthma exacerbations for the past several weeks. On review of systems he mentions that he has lost about 8 pounds over the last month. On physical exam he appears to be a healthy young man with no apparent physical anomalies. You order a UA and you find **2+ blood** without any nitrates or leukocytes.

Disease: Churg-Strauss

Pathology: Immune-mediated inflammation → immune complex deposition → idiopathic multisystem granulomatosis and vasculitis of small- and medium-sized arteries.

Characteristics: Malaise; fever; weight loss; hypertension; **hemoptysis;** melena; **hematuria;** proteinuria; abdominal pain/discomfort; muscle pain or weakness; skin lesions; **asthma.**

Diagnosis: Chest x-ray showing transient infiltrates; biopsy showing fibrin and **eosinophilic** infiltrate, **pANCA.** Can be part of polyarteritis nodosa.

Treatment: Corticosteroids; cyclophosphamide.

CARDIOLOGY—cont'd

History of Present Illness: A 58-year-man is brought into the office by his wife. She informs you that her husband has had increasing problems with **shortness of breath** while walking. He used to be quite active, but for the past 10 years has put on a considerable amount of **weight** and does not exercise any more. On physical exam his blood pressure is **180/93.** He is overweight. On cardiac exam you note a third heart sound and an elevated **JVD** (8 cm).

Disease: Congestive Heart Failure

Pathology: ↑ preload (end-diastolic volume)/ ↓ contractility/ ↑ afterload (resistance) → ↑ sympathetic activity (↑ heart rate, contractility, resistance) → cardiomegaly, pulmonary edema, liver congestion (Fig. 1.4).

Characteristics: Shortness of breath; dependent bilateral **edema;** orthopnea; paroxysmal nocturnal dyspnea. History of cardiac ischemia or arrhythmias.

Diagnosis: Clinical diagnosis; tachycardia; ↑ JVD; third heart sound; bilateral lower lobar rales; hepatomegaly; catheterization; ↑ BUN/creatinine; echocardiogram; EKG; x-ray (cardiomegaly, interstitial edema of lung); radionucleoside angiography; cardiac catheterization.

Treatment: Decrease weight, low-sodium diet, diuretics; ACE inhibitors; digoxin; hydralazine, α-blockers; β-blockers; nitrate; antiarrhythmics.

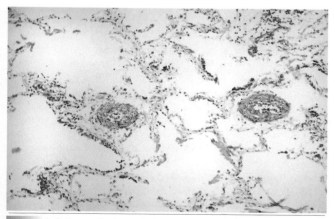

FIGURE 1.4 Congestive heart failure. © *Barry R. DeYoung, MD, University of Iowa College of Medicine.*

CARDIOLOGY—cont'd

History of Present Illness: An 8-year-old white female presents with a rash over her buttocks and thighs. Her past medical history is only significant for a mild **cold** with a fever and **abdominal pain** several days ago. On physical exam you note palpable **purpura over her buttocks and lower extremities.** While examining her she cries out in pain as you lift her knee. Both her knees are tender and swollen to palpation.

Disease: Henoch-Schönlein Purpura

Pathology: Unknown etiology?? → **IgA** immune vasculitis due to IgA immune complex deposition.

Characteristics: Children; palpable purpuric skin lesions (mostly lower extremities); edema; abdominal pain; vomiting; nonmigratory **arthralgia;** polyarthralgia; hematuria. Associated with **URI.**

Diagnosis: ↑ sedimentation rate; biopsy showing IgA in the mesangium and in crescents (glomerular nephritis).

Treatment: None because self-limited; immunoglobulin for progressive nephritis.

♦   ♦   ♦

History of Present Illness: A 30-year-old **African American** male comes in for his annual checkup. He has no previous diseases or health history. His review of systems is only positive for occasional **headaches.** On physical exam your nurse circled his blood pressure **160/97.** Otherwise his physical exam is unremarkable.

Disease: Hypertension

Pathology: ↑ pressure → left ventricular hypertrophy/myocyte hypertrophy → fibrosis → ↓ compliance → ↓ diastolic/ ↑ O_2 demand → ischemia. Primary hypertension is due to unknown etiology, but believed to be due to the interaction between genetics and environment. Secondary hypertension is due to known causes of increased blood pressure (i.e., renal disease, endocrine disorders, medication).

Characteristics: African American males increased risk. Nausea; vomiting; headache; visual changes; **paroxysmal nocturnal dyspnea;** myocardial ischemia.

Diagnosis: Clinical diagnosis; ↑ blood pressure; ↑ BUN/creatinine; chest x-ray showing left ventricular hypertrophy; hematuria and proteinuria.

Treatment: Weight loss; sodium-restricted diet; diuretics; ACE inhibitors; hydralazine, α-blockers; β-blockers; nitrate.

History of Present Illness: A 2-year-old **Asian** boy presents with fever and a red rash on his hands. His mother does not recall him touching anything toxic or injuring himself recently. He is not on any medications and has no known medical allergies. On HEENT exam you note that he has **conjunctivitis** and **cervical lymphadenopathy.** He also has **erythematous palms and soles.**

Disease: Kawasaki's Disease (AKA Mucocutaneous Lymph Node Syndrome)
Pathology: Unknown etiology. One theory is that autoantibodies to endothelial and smooth muscle cells lead to acute necrotizing vasculitis of large, medium, and small arteries.
Characteristics: Fever; erythema and **desquamation of palms and soles; conjunctivitis;** oral erythema (**"strawberry tongue"**); **cervical lymphadenopathy;** aneurysm; myocardial infarction; sudden death. Increased incidence in **Mormons** and **Asians.**
Diagnosis: Clinical diagnosis; leukocytosis; increased CRP.
Treatment: Self-limited; aspirin; IV immunoglobulin; warfarin for aneurysms.

◆   ◆   ◆

History of Present Illness: A 57-year-old **woman** presents to her physician with a chief complaint of **chest pain** and dyspnea. On review of systems she also is fatigued. Physical exam reveals no gross abnormalities. Her cardiac exam is significant for a **midsystolic click** and a **systolic murmur** that changes with position.

Disease: Mitral Valve Insufficiency
Pathology: Myxomatous degeneration **(mitral valve prolapse);** valve perforation (endocarditis); valvular dysfunction; rheumatic heart disease; cardiac tumors → **mitral valve insufficiency.**
Characteristics: Can be asymptomatic for years. Dyspnea; tachypnea; angina; CHF; **pansystolic murmur** at the apex that radiates to the axilla; **midsystolic click;** brisk carotid upstroke; hyperdynamic left ventricular impulse; death. Increased risk for **atrial fibrillation.** Associated with **Marfan's** syndrome and embolic stroke.
Diagnosis: EKG left atrial abnormality or atrial fibrillation with left ventricular hypertrophy; echocardiogram; Doppler; transesophageal echocardiogram; MRI measurement of left ventricular function; cardiac catheterization; angiography; x-ray with left atrial and ventricular enlargement.
Treatment: Intra-aortic balloon (acute stabilization); valve repair; valve replacement.

History of Present Illness: A 38-year-old **woman** presents to her family physician with fever, malaise, and abdominal pain for the past month and a half. She also notes that for the past week she has had increasing pain in her knees **(arthralgias).** On physical exam you note some purpura on her lower extremities. She also points out **painful palpable nodules** on her shins.

Disease: Polyarteritis Nodosa

Pathology: Immune complex formation **(pANCA)** → inflammation of small and medium arteries (frequently mesenteric, heart, and brain) → destruction of medial and internal elastic lamella → aneurismal nodules.

Characteristics: Fever; weight loss; nausea; vomiting; **arthralgias;** myalgias; arthritis; ischemic heart disease; abdominal pain; headache; **palpable painful nodules.**

Diagnosis: Clinical diagnosis; biopsy (gold standard); ↑ sedimentation rate; anemia; leukocytosis; **pANCA; hepatitis B** or C; angiography.

Treatment: Corticosteroids; immunosuppressive medications; cyclophosphamide.

History of Present Illness: A 22-year-old man presents with a syncopal episode this morning not associated with a bowel movement. His past medical history is only significant for having **tonsillitis** 3 weeks ago. Review of systems reveals that he has had some increasing dyspnea on exertion. On physical exam he appears to be a healthy, well-developed male in no acute distress. On auscultation you note a **diastolic murmur** at the apex.

Disease: Rheumatic Heart Disease

Pathology: Group A β-hemolytic streptococcus infection → erythematic and verrucae along high pressure cardiac valves (mitral and aortic > pulmonary and tricuspid) → fibrotic healing of valves → stenosis and valvular insufficiency. Rheumatic heart disease is a sequela of rheumatic fever. **Rheumatic fever** is an acute, immune response following infection with group A β-hemolytic strep that results in the following:
1. **P**olyarthritis
2. **E**rythema marginatum
3. **C**arditis
4. sub**C**utaneous nodules
5. **S**ydenhams chorea **(PECCS)**

Diagnosis is made by <u>Jones Criteria,</u> which is group A β-hemolytic strep infection plus one major criteria (PECCS) and two minor (fever, ↑ ESR, etc).

Characteristics: History of rheumatic fever (60%). Endocarditis results following dental, urologic, and other surgical procedures.

Diagnosis: Clinical diagnosis; echocardiogram revealing hypertrophy and mitral stenosis; EKG with an arrhythmias (atrial fibrillation common).

Treatment: Antibiotic prophylaxis; anticoagulation; prosthetic valves; antiarrhythmics.

CARDIOLOGY—cont'd

History of Present Illness: A 30-year-old **Asian woman** presents to her family physician for her annual checkup. Her only complaint is occasional changes in her **vision.** When taking her vitals you notice that she does not have any radial pulse on her left arm and a **barely palpable pulse** on the right. On physical exam she appears to be healthy.

Disease: Takayasu's Arteritis (AKA Pulseless Disease)

Pathology: Unknown etiology → granulomatous vasculitis of the medium and large arteries (common in the branches of the **aorta = Aortic Arch Syndrome**) → stenosis of the arteries.

Characteristics: Fever; night sweats; **low blood pressure in upper extremities;** coldness or numbness of the fingers; **visual disturbances;** blindness; retinal hemorrhages; dizziness; claudication of the legs. Increased incidence in **Asian** women.

Diagnosis: Absent upper pulses; angiography; biopsy showing inflammatory infiltrate (similar to giant cell arteritis).

Treatment: Corticosteroids; arterial grafts.

◆   ◆   ◆

History of Present Illness: A 53-year-old male presents to his physician for a "cold." He has a **cough** and has felt tired for the past few weeks. He has also had a **severe headache.** He reports that it comes and goes. It is not associated with any stimulus and does not respond to NSAIDs. It is a throbbing pain that shoots from his left eye up into his temple. On physical exam you note that his left **jaw is tender** to the touch. You also palpate a cord-like feel to his left temporal artery.

Disease: Temporal Arteritis (AKA Giant cell arteritis)

Pathology: Unknown etiology → autoimmune attack against the arterial wall (preferentially **temporal artery and other branches of the carotid artery**) → granuloma formation involving mononuclear cells, neutrophils, and eosinophils → can lead to systemic vasculitis and **loss of vision.**

Characteristics: Older (>50 yrs); weight loss; fatigue; fever; headache; **jaw/face pain; diplopia;** loss of vision. Associated with **polymyalgia rheumatica.**

Diagnosis: Clinical diagnosis (asymmetrical pulses); murmur or bruits, ↑ **sedimentation rate; temporal artery biopsy** (gold standard) showing lymphocytes, histiocytes, plasma cells, and **giant cells.**

Treatment: Prednisone

History of Present Illness: A 30-year-old male presents with increasing **pain in his calf** when he walks. His history is only significant for an 18-pack year history of **smoking.** On physical exam you note that his feet are dusky in color and his right pedal **pulse is absent.** There is little hair growth on his ankles and toes as well.

Disease: Thromboangiitis Obliterans (AKA Buerger's)

Pathology: Segmental vasculitis of small and medium arteries of extremities (radial and tibial common) → ischemia → microabscess and gangrene.

Characteristics: Intermittent **claudication;** palpable painful arteries; pallor; cyanosis; ulcerations/gangrene; Raynaud's. Common in **smokers** and more often in men from the Jewish population.

Diagnosis: Clinical diagnosis; angiography; HLA-B5 common.

Treatment: Discontinue smoking; sympathectomy; amputation of affected appendage.

◆　　　◆　　　◆

History of Present Illness: A 23-year-old male presents complaining of **ataxia.** He mentions that he cannot tell if it is due to the **visual changes** that he has noted recently. His past medical history is non-contributory. His family history includes a grandfather that died of **renal cell carcinoma.** On physical exam it is noted that he has some mild nystagmus and **retinal hemorrhages.**

Disease: Von Hippel-Lindau Disease

Pathology: Autosomal-dominant defect related to *ras*-oncogene on **chrom** 3p25–26 → defective production of protein pVHL → disinhibition of RNA synthesis → **hemangioblastomas** of **cerebellum, retina, brainstem, and spinal cord** and cysts in pancreas, liver, and kidneys.

Characteristics: Cerebellar ataxia, nystagmus, **retinal hemangiomas,** papilledema, dysdiadochokinesia. Increased risk of **renal cell carcinoma.**

Diagnosis: Head CT/MRI with solid or cystic lesions; abdominal CT shows renal, hepatic, or pancreatic cysts.

Treatment: Surgical removal; photocoagulation of retinal hemorrhages; partial nephrectomy of renal cell carcinomas.

CHAPTER 2
DERMATOLOGY

Disease: Acne Vulgaris

Pathology: Plugged follicles → retention of sebum → +/− infection of *Propioniobacterium acnes* → breakdown of sebaceous oils by lipases → inflammation. Endocrine may play a role, especially in adolescents.

Characteristics: Pink and purple pimply pustules; **comedones** (open or closed); erythema, scars, or open excoriations (Fig. 2.1).

Diagnosis: Clinical diagnosis.

Treatment: Retinoids; benzoyl peroxide; topical or oral antibiotics.

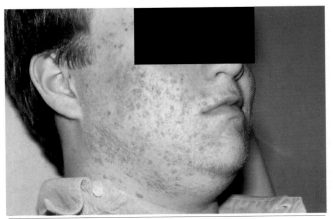

FIGURE 2.1 Acne vulgaris. © *Mary Stone, MD, University of Iowa College of Medicine.*

DERMATOLOGY—cont'd

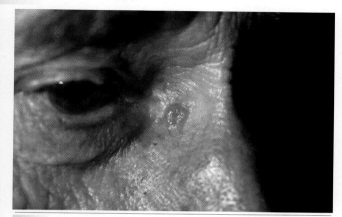

FIGURE 2.2 Basal cell carcinoma. © *Mary Stone, MD, University of Iowa College of Medicine.*

Disease: Basal Cell Carcinoma

Pathology: Basal cell hyperplasia and atypia (decreased cytoplasm and palisading basal cells) → thickened epidermis. Slow growing and rarely metastasizes.

Characteristics: Common in **sun-exposed** areas. Raised **"pearly" papule** with a raised border and telangiectatic vessels. Can ulcerate. Morpheaform basal cell carcinoma is more flat and has more irregular borders (Fig. 2.2).

Diagnosis: Clinical diagnosis with biopsy confirmation.

Treatment: Cryotherapy; fluoracil; surgical excision.

◆ ◆ ◆

Disease: Bullous Pemphigoid

Pathology: Antibody-antigen interaction (Bullous pemphigoid antigen 1 and 2) → immunoglobulin (IgG and C3) deposits at the dermoepidermal junction.

Characteristics: Tense blisters on a normal to erythematous/urticarial skin; **flexure** areas such as the thighs, groin, axillae; **oral.** More common in the elderly (Fig. 2.3).

Diagnosis: Clinical diagnosis; negative Nikolsky's; direct immunofluorescence with IgG and C3 in a **linear band at the dermoepidermal junction;** serum anti-basement membrane antibodies.

Treatment: Oral prednisone; tetracycline; nicotinamide; azathioprine; dapsone.

DERMATOLOGY—cont'd

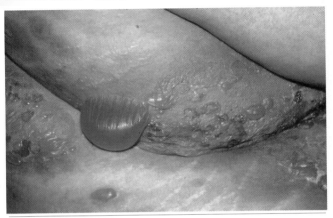

FIGURE 2.3 Bullous pemphigoid. © *Mary Stone, MD, University of Iowa College of Medicine.*

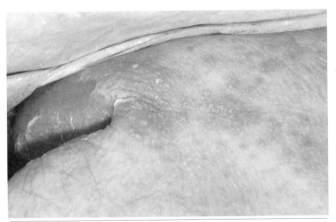

FIGURE 2.4 Candida. © *Mary Stone, MD, University of Iowa College of Medicine.*

Disease: Candida

Pathology: Normal opportunistic fungal flora of the skin, mouth, and gastrointestinal tract → pseudohyphae, true hyphae, and septa.

Characteristics: Red patches with satellite pustules ("beefy red"); thrush (white carpet) when oral, white superficial discharge on an erythematous skin when vaginal; intertriginous areas; moist areas. Associated with **diabetes,** obesity, antibiotic use, and **immunocompromised** (burn patients, AIDS, cancer) (Fig. 2.4).

Diagnosis: Clinical diagnosis; KOH; culture.

Treatment: Topical imidazoles; oral azoles; nystatin.

DERMATOLOGY—cont'd

Disease: Dermatitis Herpetiformis

Pathology: Unknown etiology/associated with **HLA-B8** and DR3 →
neutrophilic infiltrate along dermal papillae → pruritic papules.

Characteristics: Males > females. Bilateral symmetrical pruritic
grouped lesions; 3–4th decade; elbows; knee; shoulder; scalp; buttocks. Associated with gluten-sensitive enteropathy **(celiac disease).**
Increased risk of gastrointestinal lymphoma (Fig. 2.5).

Diagnosis: Clinical diagnosis; biopsy with light microscopy showing **dermal papillae** that have neutrophilic abscesses; circulating or
immunofluorescence studies showing IgA; circulating anti-
endomysium antibodies.

Treatment: Dapsone; Sulfapyradine; gluten-free diet.

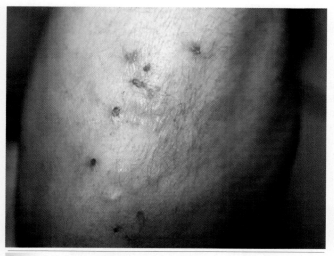

FIGURE 2.5 Dermatitis herpetiformis. © *Mary Stone, MD, University of
Iowa College of Medicine.*

DERMATOLOGY

Dermatology—cont'd

Disease: Dermatitis/Eczema

Pathology:
1. Contact dermatitis due to exposure to antigens resulting in a delayed hypersensitivity reaction
2. Atopic dermatitis has an unknown etiology
3. Drug-related dermatitis due to iatrogenic exposure to antigens
4. Photoeczematous dermatitis
5. Primary irritant dermatitis due to repeated trauma to the skin

Characteristics: Dry, white, flaky **pruritic** patches; **lichenification;** perioral; flexures (wrists, hands, neck). Positive family history for dermatitis or **asthma.**

Diagnosis: Clinical diagnosis.

Treatment: Moisturizers; topical steroids; topical tar preparations.

◆   ◆   ◆

Disease: Erythema Multiforme

Pathology: Hypersensitivity response to infections (e.g., herpes simplex), medications, malignancies, or collagen vascular diseases (lupus, dermatomyositis). In its severest drug-related form it is called **Stevens-Johnson syndrome.**

Characteristics: Target lesions; bullae occasionally, but can be macular, papular, or urticarial; common on the palms, soles, mouth, face, back, genital, and knees. Males > females; young people. **Self-limited to approximately 24 hours** (Fig. 2.6).

Diagnosis: Clinical diagnosis.

Treatment: Supportive; systemic corticosteroids.

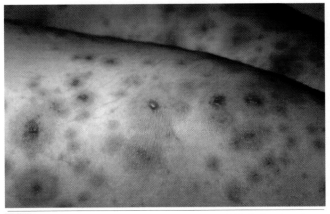

Figure 2.6 Erythema multiforme. © *Mary Stone, MD, University of Iowa College of Medicine.*

DERMATOLOGY—cont'd

Disease: Folliculitis/Furuncles/Carbuncles

Pathology: Infection (***Staph aureus;*** *pseudomonas aeroginosa.* Gram-negative, pityrosporum) of hair follicle → papules, pustules, erosion → crusting.

Characteristics: Pruritic; tender; crusty lesions; lymphadenitis.

Diagnosis: Clinical diagnosis; Gram culture.

Treatment: Topical antibacterial soap; mupirocin; oral antibiotics.

◆   ◆   ◆

Disease: Herpes Simplex

Pathology: Herpes infection (HSV 1, HSV 2) → viral replication in the skin and mucous membranes → can infiltrate the neurons → vesicular lesions.

Characteristics: Grouped vesicles; common at the **vermilion border** of the lip and genitalia (Fig. 2.7).

Diagnosis: Clinical diagnosis; Tzanck smear; culture; direct biopsy; fluorescent antigen.

Treatment: Acyclovir.

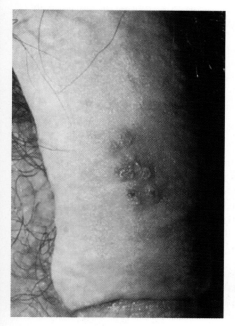

FIGURE 2.7
Herpes simplex. © *Mary Stone, MD, University of Iowa College of Medicine.*

DERMATOLOGY—cont'd

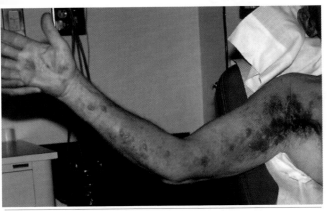

FIGURE 2.8 Herpes zoster. © Mary Stone, MD, University of Iowa College of Medicine.

Disease: Herpes Zoster

Pathology: Herpes infection (see above) → resolution of active lesion → herpes resides in nerve ganglion → erupts, frequently when **immuno-compromised.**

Characteristics: Grouped vesicles along a **dermatome;** severe pain (Fig. 2.8).

Diagnosis: Clinical diagnosis; Tzanck smear; culture; direct biopsy; fluorescent antigen.

Treatment: Acyclovir; analgesics for pain.

◆   ◆   ◆

Disease: Impetigo

Pathology: *Staphylococci* or *streptococci* infection.

Characteristics: Erythematous macules commonly on the hands and face → vesicles → **honey-colored crust** after vesicles break. Common in **children** or adults in poor health or living situations (Fig. 2.9).

Diagnosis: Clinical diagnosis; Gram stain; culture.

Treatment: Mupirocin; oral antibiotics.

◆   ◆   ◆

Disease: Inherited Epidermolysis Bullosa

Pathology: (1) EB Simplex—mutation on keratins 5 or 14; (2) Junctional EB—mutations at laminin 5, epiligrin, nicein, BPAg2; and α6β4 integrin; (3) Dystrophic EB—defect in type VII collagen.

Characteristics: Bullous lesions; shears on pressure points (hands, feet, skin, mucosa) (Fig. 2.10).

Diagnosis: Clinical diagnosis.

Treatment: Supportive.

DERMATOLOGY—cont'd

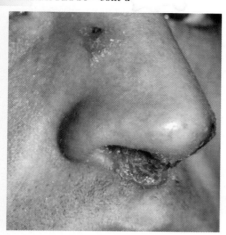

FIGURE 2.9
Impetigo. © Mary Stone, MD,
University of Iowa College of
Medicine.

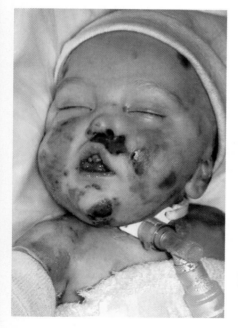

FIGURE 2.10
Inherited epidermolysis bullosa.
© Mary Stone, MD, University of
Iowa College of Medicine.

Dermatology—cont'd

Disease: Lichen Planus

Pathology: Etiology unknown?? **Lymphocytic infiltrate** in upper dermis.

Characteristics: Purple polygonal papules (cobblestone-like); pruritus (especially at wrists and ankles); Koebner phenomenon; **Wickham striae** (tiny white dots and lines over papules); ulcerations. Associated with **Hep C.** Self-limited (Fig. 2.11).

Diagnosis: Clinical diagnosis.

Treatment: Topical steroids; retinoids; PUVA.

♦   ♦   ♦

Disease: Melanoma

Pathology: Sun exposure, hereditary factors, and carcinogen exposure impact → atypical pigmented cells with irregular nuclei → horizontal and radial growth into the epidermis → depth determines tumor progression and malignancy. **Metastasis** common. Subtypes include: lentigo maligna, superficial spreading malignant melanoma, nodular melanoma, acral-lentiginous melanoma, and mucous membrane melanomas.

Characteristics: Most common cause of death related to skin disease. Change/irregularities in color, size, shape, border, or texture of a pigmented lesion. **"ABCD" (Asymmetry, Border, Color, Diameter)** Growth of a new lesion with irregular characteristics. Pruritus can occur (Fig. 2.12).

Diagnosis: Clinical diagnosis; biopsy. Breslow's classification used to predict survival: <0.67 mm; 0.76–1.69 mm; >1.69 mm.

Treatment: Surgical excision.

♦   ♦   ♦

Disease: Molluscum Contagiosum

Pathology: Viral infection by the **poxvirus** via direct contact.

Characteristics: Single or multiple firm **dimpled skin colored papules;** nodules with keratotic plug. Common on the face, hands, genitals, and lower abdomen. Associated with AIDS patients.

Diagnosis: Clinical diagnosis; biopsy showing molluscum bodies.

Treatment: Curettage; electrocautery; cryotherapy.

DERMATOLOGY—cont'd

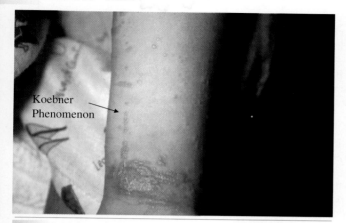

FIGURE 2.11 Lichen planus. © *Mary Stone, MD, University of Iowa College of Medicine.*

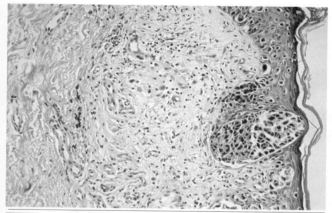

FIGURE 2.12 Melanoma. © *Barry R. DeYoung, MD, University of Iowa College of Medicine.*

DERMATOLOGY—cont'd

Disease: Pediculosis

Pathology: Infection with parasites. (1) <u>Pubic pediculosis</u>—*Pthirus pubis;* (2) <u>Pediculosis corporis</u>—*Pediculus humanus;* (3) <u>Pediculosis capitis</u>—*Pediculus humanus* var **capitis.**

Characteristics: Pruritus with excoriation; eggs in hair or on clothes.

Diagnosis: Clinical diagnosis.

Treatment: NIX; RID; permethrin rinse; lindane; nit removal.

◆   ◆   ◆

Disease: Pemphigus Vulgaris

Pathology: Autoantibody production to adhesion molecules, Desmoglein → acantholysis → bullae. Can be induced by penicillamine or captopril. Several other forms of pemphigus include *Pemphigus foliaceus, paraneoplastic pemphigus, pemphigus erythamatosus,* and *pemphigus vegetans.*

Characteristics: Flaccid blisters on the scalp, face, axilla, groin, trunk, or mouth → rupture → denuded skin; positive **Nikolsky's** sign; mid-late in life (Fig. 2.13).

Diagnosis: Clinical diagnosis; biopsy with direct immunofluorescence showing separation of epidermal cells **(acantholysis)** with **IgG;** indirect antigen showing Desmogelein 3.

Treatment: Steroids; Azathioprine; cyclophosphamide; methotrexate; chlorambucil; gold.

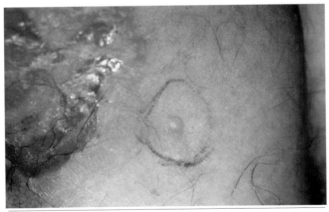

FIGURE 2.13 Pemphigus vulgaris. © *Mary Stone, MD, University of Iowa College of Medicine.*

DERMATOLOGY—cont'd

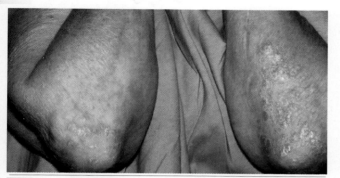

FIGURE 2.14 Psoriasis. © *Mary Stone, MD, University of Iowa College of Medicine.*

Disease: Psoriasis

Pathology: Unknown etiology. Most likely has a genetic component associated with HLA types leading to a thickened stratum corneum, Munro's microabscesses (intra/subcorneal PMNs), parakeratosis, and inflammatory infiltrate.

Characteristics: Salmon colored plaques; white scales; desquamation; **Koebner** phenomena (new lesions at site of trauma); acantholysis; mild pruritus. May be associated with arthritis, spondylitic heart disease, and myopathy (Fig. 2.14).

Diagnosis: Clinical diagnosis.

Treatment: Emollients; topical steroids; topical retinoids; calciotriene; tar; UVB; PUVA; methotrexate; acitretin; cyclosporin.

♦   ♦   ♦

Disease: Rosacea

Pathology: Unknown etiology?? → erythema, telangiectasis, and glandular hyperplasia. Can have an acneform component as well.

Characteristics: Central facial erythema; papules. Can be associated with **migraine** headaches.

Diagnosis: Clinical diagnosis.

Treatment: Topical metronidazole; systemic tetracycline or erythromycin; laser surgery for telangiectasia.

DERMATOLOGY—cont'd

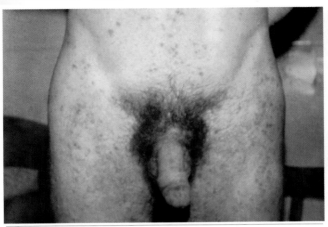

FIGURE 2.15 Scabies. © Mary Stone, MD, University of Iowa College of Medicine.

Disease: Scabies
Pathology: Infection with *Sarcoptes scabiei* → creates burrows under the stratum corneum.
Characteristics: Linear streaks on the skin. Common in the axilla, genitalia, knees, ankles, and feet (Fig. 2.15).
Diagnosis: Clinical diagnosis; mites visualized.
Treatment: Permethrin; lindane lotion/shampoo; invermectin; antihistamines; wash sheets and other possible contaminates.

♦   ♦   ♦

Disease: Syphilis
Pathology: Infection with *Treponema pallidum* (spirochete) most often through sexual contact, but can be through pregnancy → binding of spirochetes to endothelial cells → mononuclear infiltrates → antibody response.
Characteristics: <u>Primary stage</u> (approximately 3 weeks)—primary **chancre** and lymphadenopathy; <u>Latent phase</u> (of variable length) symptom free; <u>Secondary stage</u> (2–10 weeks)—secondary skin rashes, lymphadenopathy, headache, arthritis; <u>Tertiary stage</u> (years)—acute inflammation of CNS, ocular, cardiovascular involvement **(Aortic aneurysms); gummas** of the bones, skin, and viscera (Figs. 2.16 and 2.17).
Diagnosis: VDRL; FTA-ABS; darkfield or immunofluorescent staining; CSF showing ↑ protein, lymphocytic pleocytosis, and + VDRL.
Treatment: Penicillin G.

DERMATOLOGY—cont'd

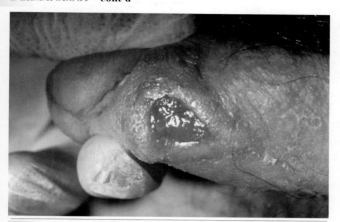

FIGURE 2.16 Syphillis. © Mary Stone, MD, University of Iowa College of Medicine.

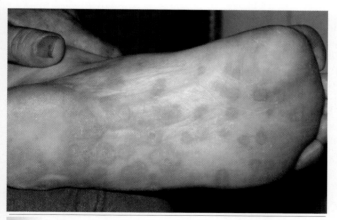

FIGURE 2.17 Syphillis. © Mary Stone, MD, University of Iowa College of Medicine.

CHAPTER 3
ENDOCRINE SYSTEM

History of Present Illness: A 34-year-old female presents with weakness, anorexia, weight loss, and diarrhea for the past few weeks. Her past medical history includes hypothyroidism. On physical exam she has **hyperpigmentation of her palmar creases** and knuckles. Her blood pressure is also low at 90/55.

Disease: Addison's Disease (Primary Adrenocortical Deficiency)

Pathology: Primary adrenal defect—most common **idiopathic** adrenal atrophy (autoimmune); infection (CMV, TB, fungal); hemorrhagic necrosis (Waterhouse-Friderichsen syndrome); metastatic carcinoma; congenital adrenal hypoplasia; pituitary failure; iatrogenic (medications).

Characteristics: Weakness; fatigue; **hypotension;** anorexia; abdominal pain; nausea and vomiting; muscle and joint pains; amenorrhea; **hyperpigmentation** (elbows, knuckles, knees, posterior neck, **palmar crease**); hypopigmentation (vitiligo); irritability; weight loss. Adrenal crisis can occur in response to stress, trauma, surgery, and infection.

Diagnosis: Neutropenia; lymphocytosis; eosinophilia, ↓ sodium; ↑ potassium; ↓ fasting blood glucose; ↓ plasma cortisol; ↑ BUN; ↑ ACTH; anti-adrenal antibodies or occasionally other antibodies. Image to rule out/in infectious causes of Addison's.

Treatment: Hydrocortisone; fludrocortisone acetate.

ENDOCRINE—cont'd

History of Present Illness: A 35-year-old **woman** presents for her annual checkup. She has no specific concerns. Her review of systems is positive for occasional **headaches** and weakness. Her physical exam is significant for a blood pressure of **193/100.**

Disease: Conn's Syndrome (Primary Aldosteronism)

Pathology: <u>Primary</u> (overproduction of mineralocorticoids)— aldosterone-secreting adenoma (AKA Conn's) (80%); hyperplasia of zona glomerulosa, carcinoma of adrenal gland; excess ACTH. <u>Secondary</u> (stimulation of renin-angiotensin)—due to renal ischemia, renal tumors, congestive heart failure, hypoalbuminemia, pregnancy.

Characteristics: Females > males. Hypertension; muscular weakness; polyuria; polydipsia; headache; parasthesias.

Diagnosis: $\uparrow$ sodium; $\downarrow$ potassium; $\downarrow$/$\uparrow$ serum renin; 24-hr urine aldosterone, cortisol, and creatinine; plasma 18-hydroxycorticosterone; $\uparrow$ plasma aldosterone.

Treatment: Surgical adrenalectomy; spironolactone (or other antihypertensives).

♦   ♦   ♦

History of Present Illness: A 28-year-old woman presents with **polyuria** and **polydipsia.** She also complains of weight gain. On physical exam you note a well-developed, slightly obese woman. Her weight is distributed in the trunk area. When you listen to her lungs, it is noticed that she has a small **hump** on her back.

Disease: Cushing's Syndrome (Hypercortisolism)

Pathology: (1) Pituitary adenoma (70%)—secretes ACTH; (2) Adrenal neoplasm—excess cortisol secretion; (3) Ectopic paraneoplastic secretion of ACTH (especially lung neoplasms); (4) Iatrogenic— ingestion of steroids $\rightarrow$ $\uparrow$ glucocorticoids.

Characteristics: Females > males. **Moon facies;** central obesity; "**buffalo hump**"; muscle weakness/wasting; thin skin; acne; polyuria; polydipsia; hirsutism; purple striae; osteoporosis; amenorrhea; hypertension; hyperglycemia; psychiatric changes; poor wound healing.

Diagnosis: Dexamethasone/dexamethasone suppression test; 24-hr urine cortisol and creatinine; midnight serum cortisol.

Treatment: Transsphenoidal resection; resection of adrenal or other source of ACTH; hydrocortisone replacement; radiation therapy.

ENDOCRINE

History of Present Illness: A 19-year-old girl is brought into her pediatrician because her mother reports that she had a fainting spell earlier that week. The girl describes it as a sudden diaphoresis and tingling feeling. Her review of systems is significant for **polyuria** and **polydipsia**. You draw a random blood glucose, and it is 250.

Disease: Diabetes Mellitus

Pathology: <u>Type I</u>—**genetic** factors such as HLA-DR3 or HLA-DR4 alleles possibly change class II T-cell receptor recognition or antigen presentation → + **autoimmune** attack of β cells → + **environmental** factors → *reduced β-cell production of insulin.* <u>Type II</u>—genetic factors that are the result of multiple defects rather than HLA defects result in *abnormal insulin secretion* → + **environmental** factors (i.e., obesity) result in *inadequate glucose utilization and peripheral tissue insulin resistance* → *β-cell exhaustion and reduced production of insulin.*

Characteristics: Polyuria; polydipsia; weakness; fatigue; polyphagia; vision changes; peripheral neuropathy; weight loss; nocturnal enuresis.

Diagnosis: Glycosylated hemoglobin; fasting/random blood glucose.

Treatment: Dietary changes; exercise; insulin; sulfonylureas; alpha-glucosidase inhibitors; thiazolidinediones; repaglinide.

◆   ◆   ◆

History of Present Illness: A 53-year-old woman presents status post a fall with extreme pain in her right hip. Her past medical history and family history is noncontributory. On x-ray you note a fracture of her right femur with **pathologic** features. The patient mentions that her right leg has been hurting her for several months. A screening panel drawn in the ER shows **hypercalcemia.**

Disease: Hyperparathyroidism

Pathology: <u>Primary</u> (excess of parathyroid hormone)—<u>parathyroid adenoma</u> (most common), hyperplasia, carcinoma, exogenous parathyroid-like hormone secretion, MEN I. <u>Secondary</u> (hypocalcemia)—<u>renal failure</u> (most common), malabsorption syndromes, Vit D or calcium deficiency.

Characteristics: Increased in >50 years. Asymptomatic; renal stones; polyuria; hypertension; constipation; fatigue; mental changes; bone pain; peptic duodenal ulcer; **pathologic fractures.**

Diagnosis: Hypercalcemia; hypo/hyperphosphatemia; hypercalciuria; elevated alkaline phosphatase; ↑ PTH; visualization of adenoma (MRI, CT, ultrasound, Tc-99m MIBI).

Treatment: Parathyroidectomy; hydration (hypercalcemia); bisphosphonates; calcium acetate (decreases hyperphosphatemia in renal failure); propranolol (prevent cardiovascular arrhythmias in hypercalcemia).

History of Present Illness: A 38-year-old woman presents with complaints of dry eyes. She also complains about generalized **fatigue** and **diarrhea.** She has no significant past medical history. Her review of systems positive for **oliogomenorrhea.** On physical exam you notice that she has lost 10 lbs since her last visit. Also, her eyes have some mild **proptosis.**

Disease: Hyperthyroidism (Thyrotoxicosis)

Pathology (Fig. 3.1)

1. Graves' disease—thyroid-stimulating immunoglobulin (IgG) stimulates TSH
2. Toxic adenomas of the thyroid (Plummer's disease)
3. Jodbasedow disease—iodine-induced hyperthyroidism
4. Excess TSH
5. Hashimoto's thyroiditis—transient hyperthyroidism
6. Malignancy—thyroid carcinoma, trophoblastic tumors
7. Pregnancy—elevated hCG activates the TSH receptors
8. Amiodarone

Characteristics: Female > male. Tachycardia; diaphoresis; weight change (loss > gain); heat intolerance; eyelid retraction; proptosis; diplopia; irritability; fatigue; weakness; tremor; fine hair; diarrhea; menstrual abnormalities. Hypokalemic periodic paralysis in men of Asian or Native American descent with thryotoxicosis.

Diagnosis: T4; T3; TSH; CXR showing mediastiral mass

Treatment: Propranolol (Graves'); methimazole; propylthiouracil; radioactive iodine; surgical resection.

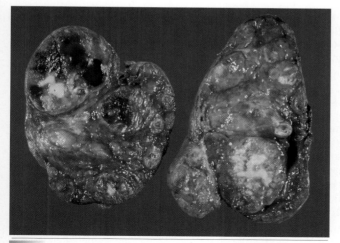

FIGURE 3.1 Hyperthyroidism/adenoma. © *Barry R. DeYoung, MD, University of Iowa College of Medicine.*

History of Present Illness: A 30-year-old woman presents with **fatigue,** lethargy, and **muscle cramps.** This has been going on for the past 4–6 months and has been getting worse. Her family history is significant for diabetes mellitus and lupus in her aunt. Review of systems is positive for **constipation** and **weight gain.** On physical exam she is noted to have **myxedema.**

Disease: Hypothyroidism

Pathology: <u>Primary hypothyroidism</u>—chronic autoimmune antithyroid antibodies **(Hashimoto thyroiditis),** iodine deficiency, thyroid enzyme defect, congenital thyroid defect, reduced thyroid functioning tissue (radiation, resection, infiltrative disorder, medically induced). <u>Secondary hypothyroidism</u>—TSH deficiency (i.e., hypopituitarism). <u>Tertiary (central) hypothyroidism</u>—TRH deficiency → ↓ thyroid hormone.

Characteristics: Female > male. **Myxedema** in adults; weakness, fatigue, cold intolerance, **constipation,** depression or other signs of mental slowness, **menorrhagia,** hoarseness, weight change (gain > loss), puffiness of eyes, hands or face, dry skin, brittle hair. **Cretinism** is hypothyroidism in infants or children. Manifests as mental retardation, short stature, umbilical hernia, protruding tongue or abdomen, or coarse facial features.

Diagnosis: ↓ free T3 or T4; ↑ increased TSH (primary); ↑ cholesterol; ↓ thyroid hormone binding ratio; ↑ antibodies against thyroperoxidase and thyroglobulin (Hashimoto's).

Treatment: Levothyroxine (thyroxine, T4).

◆   ◆   ◆

History of Present Illness: A 42-year-old man presents to his physician complaining of **palpitations** and episodes of **diaphoresis.** He also complains of **abdominal pain** and cramping. On physical exam you note that he has long arms and legs. He also has a slightly protruding tongue and bumpy lips.

Disease: Multiple Endocrine Neoplasia (MEN)

Pathology: Familial disease associated with neoplasms of multiple endocrine organs. (1) <u>MEN I</u>—parathyroid, pancreas, and pituitary neoplasms; (2) <u>MEN II A</u>—pheochromocytoma, medullary carcinoma, and parathyroid hyperplasia; (3) <u>MEN II B/ MEN III</u>—pheochromocytoma, medullary carcinomas, mucosal neuromas.

Characteristics: dependent on syndrome.

Diagnosis: CT/MRI; elevated hormone levels.

Treatment: Surgical removal; supportive.

ENDOCRINE—cont'd

History of Present Illness: A 14-year-old boy presents with complaints of severe **headaches.** He reports that they appear periodically and are associated with terrible **stomachaches,** diarrhea, and **diaphoresis.** He does not have any past hospitalizations or medical complications. Physical exam reveals a well-developed, appropriate for age adolescent boy. There are no physical abnormalities.

Disease: Pheochromocytoma

Pathology: Neoplasms of chromaffin cells → excess catecholamines. **"Rule of 10s" 10% extra-adrenal, 10% without hypertension, 10% extra-abdominal, 10% children, 10% familial, 10% bilateral adrenal involvement, 10% metastasize"** (Fig. 3.2).

Characteristics: Hypertension; **headache; palpitations; diaphoresis;** nausea; abdominal pain; chest pain; dyspnea; tremor; anxiety; weight loss; heat intolerance.

Diagnosis: Clinical presentation; urinary catecholamines; serum epinephrine or norepinephrine; ↑ blood pressure.

Treatment: Surgical removal; Nifedipine for hypertensive crisis; phenoxybenzamine.

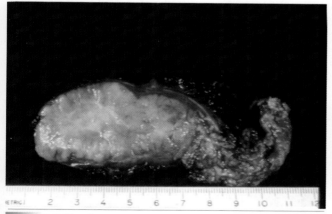

FIGURE 3.2 Pheochromocytoma. © *Barry R. DeYoung, MD, University of Iowa College of Medicine.*

CHAPTER 4
GASTROINTESTINAL

History of Present Illness: A **60**-year-old white male visits his family doctor because he has been having problems with his bowels. He says that he has colicky pain and constipation. His past medical history is significant for **polyps** removed when he was 45 years old. Other than that he has no other symptoms. On physical exam he appears well nourished in no acute distress. A bedside guaiac for him is positive.

Disease: Adenocarcinoma of the Colon

Pathology: ↓ fiber → ↑ stool bulk/ ↑ transit time in bowel → ↑ exposure to toxic waste products → dysplasia and invasion of adenocarcinoma (Fig. 4.1).

Characteristics: Most common cancer of the large intestine. **Elderly** patients; history of adenomatous **polyps;** family history of colon cancer; **asymptomatic;** hematochezia; **change in bowel habits** (constipation); tenesmus; urgency; palpable mass in the abdomen.

Diagnosis: Anemia; elevated LFT; CEA; chest and abdominal x-ray (looking for mets); colonoscopy.

Treatment: Surgical resection with lymph node dissection +/− chemotherapy.

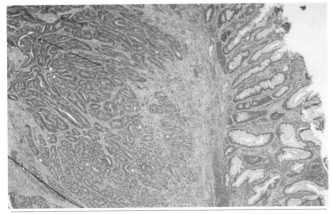

FIGURE 4.1 Adencarcinoma of the colon. © *Barry R. DeYoung, MD, University of Iowa College of Medicine.*

History of Present Illness: A 29-year-old man presents with abdominal pain and nausea. On review of systems he mentions that he has occasional **abdominal pain,** nausea, and vomiting. His past medical history is significant for **alcohol abuse,** approximately 1 pint a day. While examining him you notice that he is mildly **jaundiced** and has a liver palpable 6 cm below the costal border.

Disease: Alcoholic Hepatitis

Pathology: Alcohol abuse → macrovesicular fat, PMN infiltrate, necrosis, and **Mallory bodies** → cirrhosis.

Characteristics: Asymptomatic; hepatomegaly; **jaundice**/icterus; anorexia; nausea; vomiting; abdominal pain; splenomegaly; **ascites;** fever; encephalopathy; **Dupuytren's contractures;** palmar erythema.

Diagnosis: Clinical diagnosis; anemia on CBC; ↑ bilirubin; ↑ **AST and ALT** (AST > ALT); ↑ alkaline phosphatase; ↑ GGT; ↑ PTT; negative hepatitis A, B, C antibodies; biopsy.

Treatment: Abstinence; nutritional support; supplementary folic acid and thiamine; corticosteroid and colchicine have both been shown to have some impact in clinical studies.

♦   ♦   ♦

History of Present Illness: A 25-year-old medical student presents in the ER with severe **periumbilical pain** that radiates to the right groin region. She has been studying hard for a test and has not been eating very well for the past few days. She **vomited** two times today. Physical exam reveals a diffusely tender abdomen. She jumps off the table with deep palpation of her right lower quadrant. CBC reveals an **elevated WBC** with many neutrophils.

Disease: Appendicitis

Pathology: Inflammation or obstruction (50%–80%) of the appendix.

Characteristics: Nausea; vomiting; fever; **McBurney's** point tenderness (point between the umbilicus and iliac spine); guarding; rebound tenderness; right lower quadrant pain with hip extension **(psoas sign);** pain with internal rotation of the hip **(obturator sign).**

Diagnosis: Clinical diagnosis; **elevated WBC** with increased neutrophils; ileus or fecalith in RLQ on x-ray; US shows noncompressible tubular structure.

Treatment: Surgical removal.

GASTROINTESTINAL—cont'd

History of Present Illness: A 68-year-old man presents with a 1 year history of a cough. He attributes it to his 38-year-long **smoking** history. He also drinks heavily. He states that every time he coughs he tastes a **sour taste** in the back of his mouth. An upper GI series reveals an erythematous area at the **gastroesophageal junction.** A biopsy is sent to the laboratory for further analysis.

Disease: Barrett's Esophagitis
Pathology: Chronic reflux → metaplasia of squamous epithelium to columnar epithelium (most common at the **squamocolumnar junction**).
Characteristics: Gastroesophageal reflux disease symptoms (heartburn, regurgitation); dysphagia; can lead to severe stricture and ulcerations. **Predisposes to adenocarcinoma** (30–40 X).
Diagnosis: Clinical diagnosis; biopsy showing columnar epithelium at squamocolumnar junction.
Treatment: Cisapride; H$_2$ antagonist or other antacids; environmental changes (stop smoking; stop drinking, elevate head of bed, weight loss, decrease nocturnal food intake), follow-up observation for progression to cancer.

♦   ♦   ♦

History of Present Illness: A 37-year-old woman presents with severe **abdominal cramps** and **diarrhea.** She also mentions that she has been having "hot flashes" during which she gets flushed and feels **tachycardic.** On physical exam you find that she is slightly tachycardic and has a mild diastolic **murmur.**

Disease: Carcinoid Tumor
Pathology: Tumors of the neuroendocrine cells **(Kulchisky cells)** → release vasoactive peptides (**serotonin,** histamine, gastrin, prostaglandins).
Characteristics: Abdominal pain; diarrhea; weight loss; facial flushing; edema of the head and neck; bronchospasm; cardiac lesions; telangiectasias. Must have hepatic metastases to decrease metabolism of serotonin.
Diagnosis: Clinical diagnosis; CXR with cardiomegaly; urinary **5-hydroxyindoleacetic acid** (5-HIAA).
Treatment: Prednisone; hydration; H$_2$ receptor antagonist; octreotide; chemotherapy; surgical removal.

History of Present Illness: A 8-year-old male presents to his pediatrician for increased **diarrhea** as per mother's report. She states that his stool also has a **foul odor** to it. She says that he eats well, but that he has been **losing weight.** On physical exam you note a pale, slightly small-for-age boy. His exam is normal except for a few **vesicular lesions** on his knees.

Disease: Celiac Disease

Pathology: Gluten sensitivity (gluten is a water-insoluble protein in wheat, oat, barley, and rye) → activation of cytotoxic T cells when exposed to gluten → damage to enterocytes → blunted villi → poor absorption of nutrients.

Characteristics: Weight loss; abdominal distention; flatulence; greasy stools; **dermatitis herpetiformis;** cheilosis; ecchymoses; lactose intolerance.

Diagnosis: Physical diagnosis; CBC shows macrocytic hypochromic anemia; decreased Calcium; increased alkaline phosphatase; elevated prothrombin time; decreased serum beta-carotene; non-anion gap acidosis and hypokalemia; upper GI showing dilated jejunum; successful trial of gluten-free diet and/or gluten challenge.

Treatment: Gluten-free diet.

♦   ♦   ♦

History of Present Illness: A 45-year-old **woman** of **Native American (Pima)** heritage presents to the ER for **right upper quadrant pain.** Her review of systems is otherwise negative. Her family history is positive for cholelithiasis in all of the women in her family.

Disease: Cholelithiasis (Gallstones)

Pathology: ↑ cholesterol or calcium bilirubinate → precipitation of substances into stones.

Characteristics: Women > men; Asymptomatic; **biliary/colicky pain.** Native Americans, Crohn's disease, diabetes mellitus, rapid weight loss, and obesity are risk factors. **Increased risk of gallbladder cancer.**

Diagnosis: Radiologic (x-ray or CT); ultrasound; leukocytosis.

Treatment: Laparoscopic cholecystectomy; oral chenodeoxycholic or ursodeoxycholic acids; antibiotics.

GASTROINTESTINAL—cont'd

History of Present Illness: A 9-month-old baby boy is brought to his pediatrician. His mother is concerned because she has noticed that he is **yellow** in color. He has otherwise been healthy. On physical exam he appears to be a healthy, well-nourished, well-developed 9 month-old baby. His blood is drawn, and he is found to have a bilirubin level of 3 mg/dL.

Disease: Crigler-Najjar Syndrome

Pathology: Autosomal-recessive or -dominant defect in bilirubin UGT → absent or decreased bilirubin UGT → unconjugated hyperbilirubinemia.

Characteristics: Type I (autosomal recessive) fatal secondary to kernicterus. Type II (autosomal dominant with variable penetrance) develop jaundice +/− neurologic damage due to kernicterus.

Diagnosis: ↑ bilirubin; genetic tests; ↑ LFT; ↑ Alkaline phosphatase; liver biopsy; ultrasound; CT; MRI; ERCP. (Many of these are to rule out other causes of hyperbilirubinemia.)

Treatment: None.

◆   ◆   ◆

History of Present Illness: A 20-year-old male complains of right lower quadrant **abdominal pain** and **nonbloody diarrhea** for the past 8 months. He says that the pain is intermittent and crampy. Occasionally, he gets a fever with the diarrhea. He came in because he has lost 5 lbs over the past 2 months. Physical exam is only significant for tenderness and a **palpable mass** in the right lower quadrant.

Disease: Crohn's Disease

Pathology: Host mucosal immunity goes haywire → inflammatory bowel disease (IBD) of noncaseating granulomas with **skip lesions** and **fistulas** that run from **"mouth to anus." Systemic disease** → arthritis, **erythema nodosum,** pyoderma gangrenosum, or ankylosing spondylitis. May have a genetic component due to an increased risk in **Jewish** men.

Characteristics: Nonbloody diarrhea; abdominal pain; fever; abdominal mass in right iliac fossa; perianal fistulas or abscess; weight loss; postprandial bloating; oral aphthous lesions; musculoskeletal abnormalities (mentioned above).

Diagnosis: Barium enema—**"String sign"** or **"cobblestone"** pattern; positive guaiac; megaloblastic anemia on CBC; leukocytosis; hypoalbuminemia; ↑ ESR/CRP; negative stool cultures for bacteria or parasites.

Treatment: Dietary modification; antidiarrheal; sulfasalazine; corticosteroids; azathioprine or mercaptopurine (immunosuppressive); surgical resection or stricturoplasty.

GASTROINTESTINAL—cont'd

History of Present Illness: A 74-year-old white female in a routine nursing home checkup complains of constipation. She states that occasionally it causes her some abdominal discomfort. Physical exam only reveals mild, left lower abdominal tenderness but no mass. She has a low-grade temperature. Routine labs reveal a mild leukocytosis and decreased hemoglobin and hematocrit.

Disease: Diverticulitis

Pathology: Irritation of a blind pouch leading from the colon (food, fecal material, ulceration) (Fig. 4.2).

Characteristics: Acute abdominal pain; fever; lower abdominal tenderness/mass; constipation; pallor; **melena or gross blood per rectal exam;** nausea; vomiting.

Diagnosis: Leukocytosis; fever; ↓ hemoglobin/hematocrit; abdominal x-ray/CT may show fee abdominal air, ileus, small or large bowel obstruction. *(Flexible sigmoidoscopy and barium enemas contraindicated due to risk of perforation!)*

Treatment: Low-residue diet; metronidazole; ciprofloxacin or trimethoprim-sulfamethoxazole; surgical resection.

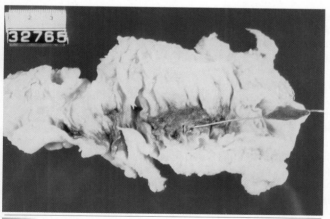

FIGURE 4.2 Diverticulitis. © *Barry R. DeYoung, MD, University of Iowa College of Medicine.*

GASTRO

GASTROINTESTINAL—cont'd

History of Present Illness: A **60-year-old African American man** complains of increasing **dysphagia** over the past year. He has more difficulties eating solid food than he does liquids. He has lost about 15 lbs over the past 3 months. Physical exam reveals supraclavicular lymphadenopathy.

Disease: Esophageal Squamous Cell Carcinoma

Pathology: Dietary and environmental factors (i.e., vitamin deficiency, ETOH, smoking, esophageal disorders).

Characteristics: Increased risk in **African Americans;** more prevalent in **>60 years;** progressive solid food **dysphagia;** weight loss; cough due to tracheobronchial extension; chest pain due to mediastinal extension; lymphadenopathy; hepatomegaly.

Diagnosis: Endoscopy with biopsy; anemia; ↑ aminotransferase; ↑ alkaline phosphatase; hypoalbuminemia; CXR shows a wide mediastinum, fistulas, pulmonary or bony metastases.

Treatment: Radiation; chemotherapy; surgical resection; combination therapy.

◆   ◆   ◆

History of Present Illness: A **63-year-old Japanese man** presents with mild anorexia and diffuse epigastric pain. His review of systems reveals that he has lost 12 lbs over the past couple of months. Physical exam is normal except for an enlarged right **supraclavicular lymph node.** His stool is guaiac positive.

Disease: Gastric Carcinoma

Pathology: *H. pylori,* low-fiber diet, low-salt diet, carcinogens (N-notroso, benzopyrene).

Characteristics: Higher incidence in Latinos, African American, Asian Americans, and those >40 years. Asymptomatic until advanced; abdominal pain; anorexia; early satiety; weight loss; vomiting; lymphadenopathy (**Virchow's** = supraclavicular; Sister Mary Joseph = umbilical); ovarian metastases (**Krukenberg cells look like signet ring cells).** Poor survival rates.

Diagnosis: Iron deficiency anemia; guaiac positive; endoscopy with biopsy; CT.

Treatment: Surgical resection; palliative combination chemotherapy (variable response rate); stent; radiation; embolization; or laser therapy for obstructions.

History of Present Illness: A 30-year-old female presents complaining of epigastric pain. She also complains of mild nausea with vomiting. Occasionally, she reports that she vomits a small amount of **dark-colored emesis.** Her past medical history is significant for **alcohol** and **tobacco** abuse. Physical exam is unremarkable as is her initial lab workup.

Disease: Gastritis

Pathology: Inflammation of the gastric mucosa: (1) Acute—due to NSAID, ETOH, smoking, uremia, stress, trauma, steroids; (2) Chronic—type A (fundal) autoimmune or type B (antral) secondary to ***Helicobacter pylori*** (90%).

Characteristics: Associated with Hashimoto's thyroiditis, gastric carcinoma; epigastric pain; nausea; vomiting; hematemesis; dyspepsia. Chronic *H. pylori* gastritis has an increased risk of **gastric adenocarcinoma** and lymphoma.

Diagnosis: ↓ hematocrit if severe bleeding; endoscopy with biopsy showing erythema, subepithelial hemorrhages, or erosions; ***H. pylori*** tests (pH test of biopsy or breath test, ELISA for IgG antibodies, QuickVue/FlexSure office-based tests).

Treatment: Sucralfate; H_2 receptor antagonists; stop offending agent use (ETOH, NSAID); antibiotics for *H. pylori*.

◆   ◆   ◆

History of Present Illness: A 28-year-old female presents to her family practice physician because of increasing **heartburn** after meals. She has noticed that when she bends down, she occasionally tastes a sour taste in the back of her throat. In the past she has taken antacids to help relieve the symptoms, but she is finding that they no longer help her discomfort. Further history-taking reveals that she used to **smoke,** but now only consumes caffeine.

Disease: Gastroesophageal Reflux Disease

Pathology: Incompetent lower esophageal sphincter or irritants (gastric reflux, **smoking**) reflux of gastric acid or contents into the esophagus → can lead to **Barrett's** esophagus.

Characteristics: heartburn; exacerbation of symptoms with reclining, bending, or large meals; cough. Increased risk if **obese** or pregnant.

Diagnosis: Clinical diagnosis; endoscopy; barium esophagography; pH monitoring (gold standard); esophageal manometry.

Treatment: Behavior modification (elevate head of bed, small meals, dietary changes); H_2 receptor antagonist; motility drugs (cisaprid and metoclopramide); surgical repair.

History of Present Illness: A 17-year-old adolescent male shows up for his sports physical. He is training for the state finals in wrestling. His coach is concerned because he says the boy looks a little pale and yellow. His past medical history and review of systems are negative. On physical exam you find a very healthy, muscular, youth. He mentions at this time that he has been working hard to lose 5 extra pounds so he can compete in the lower weight class.

Disease: Gilbert's Syndrome

Pathology: Autosomal dominant defect → decreased bilirubin UGT → unconjugated hyperbilirubinemia.

Characteristics: Benign; fluctuating jaundice that increases with **stress, illness; or exercise.**

Diagnosis: ↑ bilirubin; ↑ LFT; ↑ alkaline phosphatase; liver biopsy; ultrasound; CT; MRI; ERCP. (Many of these are to rule out other causes of hyperbilirubinemia.)

Treatment: None.

◆   ◆   ◆

History of Present Illness: A 52-year-old man complains of increasing shortness of breath with exertion. He is afraid he is having angina. Family history reveals that his father died of an MI. On physical exam you note that he is not obese, but that his skin is a dark **bronze** color as if he had a suntan. He denies visiting any tanning salons or using self-tanning creams. He mentions that he thinks that his **breasts** are increasing in size.

Disease: Hemochromatosis

Pathology: Mutation on chromosome **6** → impairs transferrin/uptake of iron → hemosidering accumulation in liver, kidney, heart, adrenals, testes, pituitary.

Characteristics: arthropathy; hepatomegaly; hepatic insufficiency; **skin pigmentation;** cardiomegaly; testicular atrophy; impotence; gynecomastia; diabetes. Increased risk of **hepatocellular carcinoma.**

Diagnosis: Clinical diagnosis; ↑ iron, transferrin, and ferritin; ↑ total iron binding capacity; ↑ glucose; ↑ AST/ALT; CT or MRI; biopsy of organ affected revealing hemosiderin infiltration; often HLA-A3 or HLA-B14 linked.

Treatment: Phlebotomy; deferoxamine; supportive treatment for any organ failure; liver transplantation.

History of Present Illness: A 10-day-old male infant has **not passed a stool** in the past 48 hours. The infant is crying constantly and has decreased feeds for the past 24 hours. The baby has vomited following the past two attempts at feeding. On exam the baby is crying and irritable. His abdomen is firm and tender to palpation.

Disease: Hirschsprung's Disease
Pathology: Failure of migration of the neural crest cells → absence of ganglionic cells in the mucosal and myenteric neural plexus → poor/absent peristalsis and **colonic dilation.**
Characteristics: Newborn presentation; constipation; abdominal distension; bowel movement on digital rectal examination; associated with **Down syndrome (10% of Hirschsprung's).**
Diagnosis: Clinical diagnosis; abdominal x-ray; CT.
Treatment: Dietary changes; osmotic laxatives; cathartic laxatives; enemas; surgical resection.

◆   ◆   ◆

History of Present Illness: A frantic mother brings in her 6-day-old **son.** He is her **first child,** and she is worried that he is not eating well. He appears to be hungry and eager to feed each time, but he does not feed for very long. The baby breast-feeds for a few minutes, and then he **vomits.** On abdominal exam you palpate a small **knot** near the baby's stomach.

Disease: Hypertrophic Pyloric Stenosis
Pathology: Abnormal thickening of the pylorus.
Characteristics: Males more frequently than females; **first born males;** vomiting; poor feeding; weight loss; palpable **"olive"** of the pyloric sphincter.
Diagnosis: Clinical diagnosis; barium study; x-ray.
Treatment: Surgical valvoplasty.

◆   ◆   ◆

History of Present Illness: A 1-month-old male infant is brought in for his 1-month, well-child care check. His mother says that he has been healthy without any infections. While plotting out his height and weight, you notice that he is **below the 5th percentile** on the growth chart. His physical exam is otherwise normal.

Disease: Intestinal Atresia
Pathology: Failure to recanalize the lumen of the intestine.
Characteristics: Associated highly with **Down** syndrome and VATER (**V**ertebral, **A**nal atresia, **T**racheoesophageal atresia, **R**enal dysplasia).
Diagnosis: CXR = **"double bubble"** in duodenal atresia.
Treatment: Surgical intervention.

Gastrointestinal—cont'd

History of Present Illness: A 51-year-old man presents with a 6-month history of **intermittent vomiting.** He states that he has had no change in his diet. His bowel movements are normal. Occasionally, he has noticed streaks of **blood** in his vomitus. He states that there is increasingly more blood in the vomit. His past medical history is significant for tobacco and **ETOH abuse.**

Disease: Mallory-Weiss Syndrome

Pathology: Longitudinal tears in the esophagus due to excessive vomiting, retching, and reflux (Fig. 4.3).

Characteristics: Boerhaave's syndrome; bloody vomitus; retching; associated with **ETOH** abuse.

Diagnosis: Clinical diagnosis; endoscopy; biopsy to rule out neoplasm.

Treatment: Stop offending agent; transfuse; octreotide; intra-arterial embolization.

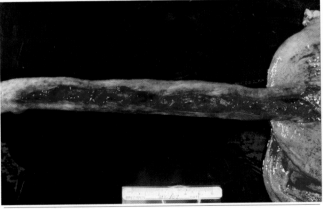

Figure 4.3 Mallory-Weiss syndrome. © *Barry R. DeYoung, MD, University of Iowa College of Medicine.*

History of Present Illness: A **2-year-old boy** presents to his pediatrician. His mother reports that he has had three red diapers recently **(hematochezia).** He does not complain of any pain. His mother cannot see or palpate any lesions around his anus. On physical exam he appears to be slightly pale. His is mildly **tachycardic.** On abdominal exam you note that he has a **distended** abdomen. Digital rectal exam is positive for **occult blood.**

Disease: Meckel's Diverticulum

Pathology: Persistence of the vitelline duct → diverticulum from the ileum. *Most common congenital GI abnormality.*

Characteristics: Melena; hematochezia, abdominal pain; **abdominal distension,** tachycardia. **Rule of 2's: 2% of population, 2 inches long, 2 years old, 2 feet from ileocecal valve, 2 types of epithelium (gastric and pancreatic).**

Diagnosis: CBC, anemia, leukocytosis, electrolytes, hemeoccult.

Treatment: Surgical correction, fluid management.

◆   ◆   ◆

History of Present Illness: A 62-year-old white male presents to the local VA for **nausea** and vomiting. His review of systems is also positive for **anorexia.** His past medical history is significant for a long history of **alcohol abuse.** On physical exam you note he has abdominal pain and tenderness. His temperature is mildly elevated.

Disease: Pancreatitis

Pathology: Inappropriate activation of pancreatic enzymes → autodigestion and damage of acinar cells.

Characteristics: Epigastric pain with radiation to the back; **nausea;** vomiting; sweating; anorexia; abdominal pain; fever; previous history of symptoms. **ETOH abuse** and **biliary disease** common.

Diagnosis: Leukocytosis; proteinuria; granular casts; glycosuria; hyperglycemia; ↑ serum bilirubin; ↑ **amylase;** ↑ **serum lipase;** "sentinel loop" or "colon cutoff sign" on x-ray; CT. *Ranson's criteria (3+ criteria predicts a more severe course) = Age >55; WBC >16,000/μL; serum glucose >200 mg/dL; LDH >350 units/L; AST >250 units/L.*

Treatment: Rest; NPO; pain control; IV fluids; laparoscopic cholecystectomy.

History of Present Illness: A 23-year-old female medical student presents to student health (AKA Student Death) with complaints of increasing abdominal pain. She states that the pain is **gnawing.** She has been too busy to try any antacids; instead, she finds that eating a few crackers helps relieve the pain. Social history reveals that she drinks **alcohol** socially and drinks caffeine excessively. Physical exam reveals mild abdominal discomfort with deep palpation.

Disease: Peptic Ulcer Disease

Pathology: Imbalance between mucosal defense or gastric acid production. ***H. pylori*** is offending agent in 70% of ulcers.

Characteristics: Chronic gastritis (85%–100%); epigastric pain; pain/discomfort relieved by food; smoking.

Diagnosis: Clinical diagnosis; rapid urease breath test; ELISA *H. pylori* antibody positive; mucosal biopsy +/− culture.

Treatment: Antibiotics; proton pump inhibitor.

◆   ◆   ◆

History of Present Illness: A 37-year-old female presents to her doctor for bright **red blood per rectum** two times in the past week. She has no other complaints. Her review of systems is negative and past medical history unremarkable. She is concerned because she has a strong **family history of polyps** and colon cancer. Physical exam is completely within normal limits.

Disease: Polyps

Pathology: A polyp is a small mass that projects into the colon or small intestine. Classified into three groups: nonneoplastic (hyperplastic, juvenile, hamartomas, inflammatory, Peutz-Jegher); adenomatous (tubular > villous, tubolovillous); and submucosal. Familial polyposis syndromes include Peutz-Jeghers, familial adenomatous (autosomal-dominant), Gardner's syndrome, and hereditary nonpolyposis colorectal cancer (HNCC).

Characteristics: Familial, asymptomatic, weakness, fatigue, hematochezia.

Diagnosis: Fecal occult; barium enema; flexible sigmoidoscopy; colonoscopy.

Treatment: Surgical removal; aspirin or other NSAIDs.

GASTROINTESTINAL—cont'd

History of Present Illness: A 29-year-old **Jewish** male presents with a recent onset of **bloody diarrhea.** He has been having increasing abdominal cramps and the urge to defecate. On physical exam you find that he has mild orthostatic hypotension and abdominal tenderness. A digital rectal exam shows gross blood.

Disease: Ulcerative Colitis

Pathology: Host mucosal immunity goes haywire → inflammatory bowel disease (IBD) of mucosal inflammation with **crypts** in the colon and rectum. Systemic disease → arthritis, **erythema nodosum,** pyoderma gangrenosum, ankylosing spondylitis, clubbing. Might have a genetic component due to increased risk in Jewish men (Fig. 4.4).

Characteristics: Bloody diarrhea +/− mucus; abdominal pain/cramps; fecal urgency; fever; weight loss; **toxic megacolon.** Extraintestinal manifestations: arthritis, iritis, episcleritis, thromboembolic events, sclerosing cholangitis erythema nodosum, pyoderma gangrenosum. Increased risk of progressive **cancer.**

Diagnosis: Sigmoidoscopy (barium enemas are not recommended due to the risk of precipitating toxic megacolon).

Treatment: Dietary modification (parenteral if necessary); antidiarrheal; mesalamine; olsalazine; sulfasalazine; hydrocortisone; methylprednisolone; surgery.

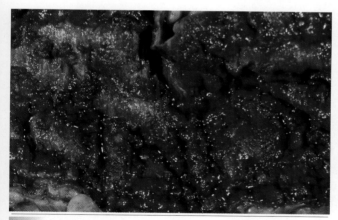

FIGURE 4.4 Ulcerative colitis. © *Barry R. DeYoung, MD, University of Iowa College of Medicine.*

GASTRO

GASTROINTESTINAL—cont'd

History of Present Illness: A 50-year-old male is brought to the local ER by his wife. She noted that recently he has been acting very strangely. She says that he is usually forgetful, but recently it has rapidly become worse. Today, she noted that he was also moving very weirdly. She said he looked like he was **writhing**. Past medical history is significant for hepatic disease. On physical exam you note mild **hepatosplenomegaly.**

Disease: Wilson's Disease

Pathology: Autosomal recessive defect on **chrom 13** → defective cooper transporting adenosine triphosphate in liver → decreased serum **ceruloplasmin** → ↓ cooper uptake → deposits in the liver, basal ganglia, and cornea **(Kayser-Fleischer ring)** (Fig. 4.5).

Characteristics: Young; liver disease; **neuropsychiatric disease** (rigidity and parkinsonian tremor common); Kayser-Fleischer rings; renal calculi; hypoparathyroidism; renal tubular acidosis.

Diagnosis: ↑ urinary cooper excretion; ↓ serum ceruloplasmin; liver biopsy.

Treatment: Dietary reduction of copper; penicillamine; zinc acetate.

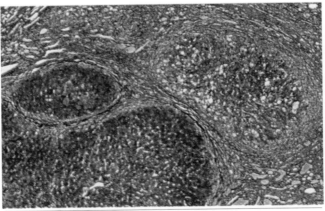

FIGURE 4.5 Wilson's disease. © *Barry R. DeYoung, MD, University of Iowa College of Medicine.*

GASTROINTESTINAL—cont'd

History of Present Illness: A 38-year-old male presents to his family
doctor for severe **diarrhea.** He has had diarrhea for the past 2 weeks.
He also complains of long-standing reflux and abdominal pain. His
past medical history includes diabetes and **peptic ulcer** disease. On
physical exam he is a well-developed, healthy appearing male. His
exam is normal except for mild **epigastric pain** on palpation. His digital rectal exam reveals occult blood.

Disease: Zollinger-Ellison Syndrome
Pathology: Gastrin-secreting tumor of the pancreas — usually, the **delta
cells** of the pancreas.
Characteristics: Recurrent peptic ulcer disease; hypergastrinemia; diar-
rhea; **MEN 1;** gastroesophageal reflux; weight loss.
Diagnosis: ↑ gastrin; ↓ gastric pH; CT/MRI; somatostatin receptor
scintigraphy; endoscopic ultrasound.
Treatment: Surgical resection; proton pump inhibitors.

CHAPTER 5
GENITOURINARY

History of Present Illness: A 58-year-old male presents with **increased frequency of urination.** He has been urinating every couple of hours for the past couple of weeks. He has also had episodes of **nocturia.** His past medical history is not positive for any major diseases. His physical exam reveals an **enlarged hard prostate.**

Disease: Benign Prostatic Hypertrophy

Pathology: Dihydrotestosterone (DHT) produced in the prostate → binds to androgen receptors → transcription of growth factors → prostatic hyperplasia.

Characteristics: Dysuria; polyuria; nocturia; difficulty starting or stopping urine stream, bladder distention/infection.

Diagnosis: Clinical diagnosis; digital rectal exam; PSA; uroflowmetry and imaging (x-ray, intravenous urography) rarely used now.

Treatment: If extreme bladder distention, suprapubic catheterization; finasteride; alpha blockers; surgical resection; antibiotics for infection.

GENITOURINARY—cont'd

History of Present Illness: A 59-year-old woman presents to her family physician for her annual pap smear. She reports no new illnesses or health problems. Her past medical history only reveals a broken leg as a child. Her physical exam reveals a small nontender palpable mass in her left breast. She does not do monthly breast exams and had not noted it before.

Disease: Breast Cancer

Pathology: Loss in cell regulation → epithelial herperplasia or sclerosing adenosis → atypical hyperplasia → progressive alterations in oncogenes, tumor suppressor genes, changes in cell structure or adhesion, increased angiogenesis, increased expression of proteases → carcinoma (Fig. 5.1).

Characteristics: Risk factors include: family history, delayed childbearing, personal history of breast cancer, nulliparity, older age. Nontender; firm mass; **skin/nipple retraction (orange peel** appearance); axillary lymphadenopathy; erythema; pain; edema/enlargment of breast.

Diagnosis: Mammogram; ultrasound; biopsy (fine-needle aspiration, large-needle aspiration, open biopsy).

Treatment: Lumpectomy +/− node resection; chemotherapy; radiation; Tamoxifen.

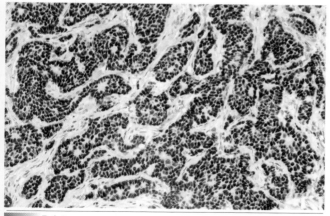

FIGURE 5.1 Breast cancer. © *Barry R. DeYoung, MD, University of Iowa College of Medicine.*

History of Present Illness: A 34-year-old woman presents to her
physician for a follow-up pap smear. She had been experiencing some
postcoital bleeding. Her last pap smear showed some cell atypia,
and she is here for her 6-month follow-up pap smear. On external
examination with the colposcopy they note some irregularities around
the endocervical junction. A biopsy is taken.

Disease: Cervical Cancer

Pathology: Sexual intercourse → human papilloma virus **(HPV)** →
koilocytotic atypia → atypia in squamous epithelium → anisokaryosis,
increased/abnormal mitotic figures, hyperchoromasia → loss of epithelial layers (Fig. 5.2).

Characteristics: Asymptomatic; postcoital bleeding; bloody discharge;
bladder or rectal dysfunction; young age at first intercourse/childbirth;
multiple sexual partners. Can be impacted by impaired immune system, smoking, or oral contraceptives.

Diagnosis: Pap smear; colposcopy +/− biopsy.

Treatment: Cauterization; cryosurgery; CO_2 laser; loop resection;

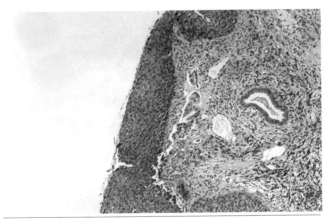

Figure 5.2 Cervical cancer. © *Barry R. DeYoung, MD, University of
Iowa College of Medicine.*

conization.

History of Present Illness: A 59-year-old **nun** presents to her physician with complaints of fatigue and weight loss. She is **obese,** without any recent weight loss. Her review of systems is significant for occasional **vaginal bleeding.** There is nothing notable on physical exam, but you draw a CBC. It reveals a hemoglobin of 9.0 g/dL.

Disease: Endometrial Carcinoma

Pathology: Unopposed estrogen → endometrial hyperplasia. Can occur in a without unopposed estrogen (Fig. 5.3).

Characteristics: >40 years, peak between 55–65 years. Asymptomatic; vaginal bleeding; weight loss; fatigue (due to anemia). Increased risk in obese, diabetic, hypertensive, late menopause, and nulliparity women.

Diagnosis: Normocytic, normochromic anemia; Pap smear showing atrophic tissue; curettage with histology.

Treatment: Surgical resection; radiation; chemotherapy.

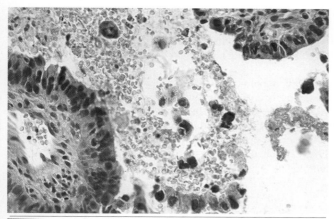

FIGURE 5.3 Endometrial carcinoma. © *Barry R. DeYoung, MD, University of Iowa College of Medicine.*

GU

History of Present Illness: A 26-year-old woman presents to her gynecologist for extremely **painful periods.** She states that she has excessive cramping associated with her periods. They have always been painful, but have been getting increasingly more painful and frequent. Nothing over-the-counter seems to help with her pain. Her review of systems reveals **dyspareunia.** Her physical exam and vaginal exam are within normal limits.

Disease: Endometriosis

Pathology: Endometrial tissue outside the uterine cavity.

Characteristics: Dysmenorrhea; dyspareunia; infertility; hypermenorrhea.

Diagnosis: Clinical diagnosis; US showing cystic masses; laparoscopy is the gold standard showing **"chocolate cysts."**

Treatment: NSAIDs; oral contraceptives; androgens; GnRH agonists; surgical treatment.

◆   ◆   ◆

History of Present Illness: A 28-year-old type I diabetic status post right kidney transplant returns for a routine checkup. Her review of systems is positive for discomfort from the multiple **autoimmune medications** she is on. Her physical exam reveals several **mobile,** nontender, rubbery, palpable masses on her left and right breasts.

Disease: Fibroadenoma of the Breast

Pathology: Benign growth of fibrous and glandular tissue.

Characteristics: Women <30 years most often. Well-circumscribed, mobile, rubbery breast mass. Mild increased risk of breast cancer. Common in women on **cyclosporin A.**

Diagnosis: Biopsy to rule out carcinoma.

Treatment: Surgical excision.

History of Present Illness: A 30-year-old G_1P_0 woman presents to her obstetrician for her 16-week checkup. She states that she has had **painless bleeding** over the past day. She also has had excessive **vomiting** for the past month. Her physical exam is significant for a fundal height of 23 cm above her umbilicus. An ultrasound is performed and reveals no fetal parts or fetal heart tones. The ultrasound has a **"snowstorm"** appearance.

Disease: Hydatidiform Mole

Pathology: (1) <u>Complete moles</u>—Fertilization of an egg that has lost its chromosomes → 90% are 46,XX (one sperm) and 10% are 46, XX and 46, XY (two sperm) → no embryonic development. (2) **Partial moles**—Fertilization of an egg with either one or two sperm → triploid (69, XXY), tetraploid (69, XYY) karyotypes → viable embryo and can produce fetal parts.

Characteristics: Presumed pregnant **with elevated** corresponding β-HCG and increasing fundal height. Abnormal uterine bleeding; abdominal pain; no fetal movement; vomiting; passage of grapelike vesicles vaginally. Increased risk of **choriocarcinoma** with complete moles.

Diagnosis: ↑↑ β-**HCG** (>**100,000**); ultrasound showing "honeycombed uterus" or **"cluster of grapes"**; ↓ serum human placental lactogen.

Treatment: Surgical removal with follow-up hCG monitoring.

◆ ◆ ◆

History of Present Illness: A 25-year-old male presents to his physician for **enlargement of his right testicle.** He reports that it is painless, but has been growing larger for the past 2 months. His review of systems is negative. On physical exam there is a firm, nontender mass on his testicle that does not illuminate. It is also noted that he has some mild **gynecomastia.**

Disease: Testicular Cancer

Pathology: (1) <u>Germ cell tumors</u> (95%)—seminoma, embryonal carcinoma, yolk sac tumor, polyembryoma, choriocarcinoma, teratomas. Can be of one histological type or multiple. (2) <u>Nongerminal/stromal tumors</u>—Leydig, sertoli, granulosa.

Characteristics: Painless mass in testis; **gynecomastia.** Risk factors include **cryptorchidism,** genetic factors, testicular dysgenesis.

Diagnosis: ↑ AFP or hCG; CXR for metastasis; US/MR tests.

Treatment: Orchiectomy; chemotherapy.

CHAPTER 6
HEMATOLOGY

History of Present Illness: A 45-year-old homosexual man presents to his physician complaining of **fatigue** and **weight loss**. He has had increasing fatigue over the past 3 months. He also reports night sweats on his review of systems. On physical exam you note that he has several light-brown skin spots on his trunk consistent with **Kaposi's sarcoma**. The remainder of the exam in within normal limits.

Disease: AIDS
Pathology: HIV gp 120 protein binds to CD4+ T cells → HIV viron enters the cells → replicates → causes cell death → ↓ humoral and cell-mediated responses → ↑ opportunistic infections and malignancies.
Characteristics: Asymptomatic, fevers, chills, weight loss, pneumonia, anorexia, nausea, vomiting, sinusitis, hairy leukoplakia, **Kaposi sarcoma.**
Diagnosis: Clinical diagnosis; HIV antibody and antigen; CD4 count.
Treatment: Prophylaxis of opportunistic diseases; antibiotics for infections; treatment for malignancies; antiretroviral therapies.

◆　　◆　　◆

History of Present Illness: A 28-year-old G_1P_0 at 24 weeks gestation presents to her obstetrician for a routine visit. She has been doing well these past few weeks and has been without any morning sickness or vaginal discharge. She does complain that she is easily **fatigued**. A physical exam is unremarkable except for **pallor.**

Disease: Anemia
Pathology: Iron deficiency; chronic disease; chronic/acute blood loss; thalassemias; Vit B12 deficiency; sideroblastic anemia; folic acid deficiency; red cell aplasia; hemolytic anemia (mechanical or immunologic); hereditary spherocytosis; paroxysmal nocturnal hemoglobinuria; glucose-6-phosphate dehydrogenase deficiency; sickle cell anemia; cold agglutin disease; hemoglobin C disorders.
Characteristics: Fatigue; tachycardia; palpitations; tachypnea; cheilosis; pallor; pica.
Diagnosis: ↓ RCB with or without morphologic abnormalities.
Treatment: Correct underlying cause (i.e., stop bleeding; Fe supplement; folic acid supplement; B12 supplement; splenectomy; etc.).

HEMATOLOGY—cont'd

History of Present Illness: A 6-month-old male presents at his well-child care checkup with **recurrent otitis media.** His mother reports that he had **bronchitis, pneumonia,** and three episodes of otitis media since his birth. On exam you note an irritable infant with a mild fever and a bulging tympanic membrane on the right.

Disease: Bruton's X-Linked Agammaglobulinemia

Pathology: Genetic mutation in tyrosine kinase (Bruton tyrosine kinase **Xq21.2–22**) → failure of pro-B cells and pre-B cells to develop into B cells. "Bruton's males BAD B-cells."

Characteristics: Recurrent bacterial and viral infections. *Haemophilus influenzae, Streptococcus pneumoniae,* or *Staphylococcus aureus* most often. Cytomegalovirus, Ebstein-Barr; and Varicella most often. *Giardia lambia* can cause intestinal distress.

Diagnosis: Clinical suspicion; ↓ B cells in serum; ↓ germinal centers throughout the body.

Treatment: IVIG.

◆   ◆   ◆

History of Present Illness: A 2-year-old boy is brought to his pediatrician for recurrent infections. His mother reports that he has always had difficulties with diaper rash. The rash is **"red and beefy"** looking. His past medical history is significant for many **recurrent infections,** both skin and respiratory. On physical exam you note a red rash with satellite pustules. They extend into his intertriginous areas.

Disease: Chronic Granulomatous Disease

Pathology: X-linked or recessive defect > decreased oxidative burst, defective NADPH oxidase due to a defect in cytochrome b, β chain.

Characteristics: Males > females. Recurrent opportunistic infections.

Diagnosis: Defective NADPH activity.

Treatment: Antibiotic treatment.

HEMATOLOGY—cont'd

History of Present Illness: A 5-year-old girl is presents with her **5th ear infection** this year. She has had a mild fever, is irritable, and has been tugging at her left ear for the past 24 hours. Her past medical history is significant for a **tonsillectomy,** pneumonia, and recurrent ear infections all her life. On physical exam she is flushed and warm to the touch. Her left ear is red, injected, and there is a loss of bony landmarks. You note that she has very fair features (albino).

Disease: Chédiak-Higashi Syndrome
Pathology: Autosomal-recessive defect in membrane-associated protein for docking and fusion → defective degranulation and pagocytosis.
Characteristics: Recurrent infections (Staph, Strep); albinism; cranial nerve and peripheral neuropathy, bleeding disorders.
Diagnosis: Neutropenia.
Treatment: Prophylactic antibiotics.

◆   ◆   ◆

History of Present Illness: A 14-year-old boy presents with recurrent sinusitis. He says his nose is congested and runny. He does not have a fever or chills. His past medical history is significant for bilateral tubes due to recurrent **otitis media, pneumonia,** and **bronchitis.** On physical exam he is in no acute respiratory distress, and his lungs are clear to auscultation. His maxillary sinuses are tender to palpation, and his right ear shows some erythema.

Disease: Common Variable Immunodeficiency
Pathology: Defective differentiation of B cells → decreased antibody-secreting plasma cells.
Characteristics: Increased or recurrent pyogenic infections; gastrointestinal infections; autoimmune cytopenia; enlarged lymph nodes; noncaseating granulomas; increased risk of carcinoma (gastric 50X risk).
Diagnosis: ↓ serum immunoglobulins; ↓ antibody production/function; normal B-cell count.
Treatment: IVIG.

History of Present Illness: A 2-month-old boy presents in the ER for an increased respiratory effort and a temperature of 102° for the past 2 days. On physical exam he is tachypneic, febrile, II/VI systolic murmur, and he has bilateral ronchi at the lower lung bases. He is microcephalic with low set ears and a small jaw.

Disease: DiGeorge's Syndrome

Pathology: Deletion on chromosome **22q11** → defective third and fourth pharyngeal pouch development → **T-cell deficiency.**

Characteristics: Recurrent infections; tetany; congenital heart defects; micrognathia.

Diagnosis: Clinical diagnosis; hypocalcemia; CT shows absence of thymus/parathyroid glands.

Treatment: Supportive; antibiotics for infection; antibiotic prophylaxis.

◆   ◆   ◆

History of Present Illness: A 34-year-old male presents in the ER after a MVA with a truck. He is bleeding from multiple sites on his upper and lower extremities. He is conscious but incoherent. His breathing is shallow and he is turning blue. On physical exam he is **hypotensive,** tachycardic, and tachypneic. It is noted that small **petechiae** are forming around his wound sites.

Disease: Disseminated Intravascular Coagulation

Pathology: Secondary complication of diseases that release tissue factor (i.e., obstetric complications, infections, neoplasms, injury, shock, liver disease, snakebite) → activation of the intrinsic and extrinsic coagulation pathways → microthrombi → activation of fibrinolysis → inhibition of platelet aggregation, thrombin, and fibrin polymerization.

Characteristics: Bleeding from oral mucosa or diathesis of the skin; respiratory distress; cyanosis; convulsions; coma; shock; oliguria; shock.

Diagnosis: Clinical diagnosis; ↓ PTT; prolonged PT or PTT; ↑ fibrin split products.

Treatment: Treatment of underlying disease/cause of DIC; anticoagulants; platelets; cryoprecipitate; aminocaproic acid.

History of Present Illness: A 3-year-old presents to the ER for severe dehydration. Her mother reports that she has been fussy and has not eaten for the past 4 days. A week ago she suffered from **bloody diarrhea** for 2 days. She also has had 2 episodes of emesis and **decreased urinary output.** On physical exam you note that she is irritable, crying, and mildly febrile. On inspection there is pallor and **periorbital edema.**

Disease: Hemolytic Uremic Syndrome

Pathology: Activation of endothelial damage (i.e., verotoxins in *E. coli*) → activated intravascular thrombosis.

Characteristics: Familial; anemia; bleeding; **renal failure**/decreased urine output; precipitated by a viral or **bacterial infection (*E. coli; shigella; salmonella*);** also precipitated by estrogen replacement therapy, postpartum, corticosteroid therapy; autologous bone marrow transplantation; immunosuppression.

Diagnosis: Clinical diagnosis; **thrombocytopenia;** hemolytic anemia without fragmented RBC; ↑ LDH; ↑ fibrin degradation products; **hyaline thrombi** in renal arterioles and glomeruli; UA with RBC casts, proteinuria, hematuria. (Normal coagulation tests, neurologic status, and Coombs'.)

Treatment: Nothing in children because it is self-limiting; plasmapheresis; fresh-frozen plasma.

◆   ◆   ◆

History of Present Illness: A 27-year-old **male** presents in the ER after an injury to his right knee while playing soccer. He recalls getting struck in the knee by another player. Since then he has been in extreme pain. On physical exam he appears to have a large **hemarthroses** on his right knee. There are no other significant physical exam findings.

Disease: Hemophilia A

Pathology: X-linked recessive trait → defective factor VIII (either decreased amount or activation) → decreased activation of the coagulation cascade.

Characteristics: Second most common bleeding disorder. Increased bleeding and bruising; **spontaneous hemarthroses; males** > females; mild bleeding disorder in heterozygous females; HIV due to transmission in transfused factor VIII.

Diagnosis: ↑ PTT; ↓ factor VIII; ↓ platelets.

Treatment: Infusion of factor VIII, desmopressin acetate.

History of Present Illness: 58-year-old man is brought into his family physician because of a weight loss (10 lbs) and fevers for the past month and a half. He has been feeling increasingly fatigued and lethargic for the past 4 months. His past medical history is unremarkable. Physical exam findings include right-sided clavicular **lymphadenopathy.**

Disease: Hodgkin's Disease

Pathology: Clonal tumor of unknown etiology. EBV hypothesized to be the cause. Categorized into lymphocytic, mixed cellularity, lymphocytic depleted, or nodular sclerosis. **Reed-Sternberg** cells (binucleate giant cells with eosinophilic nucleoli = **"owl eye cells"**) are pathonomonic (Fig. 6.1).

Characteristics: Bimodal distribution in 20s and 50s; **painless contiguous lymphadenopathy;** fever; night sweats; weight loss; splenomegaly.

Diagnosis: CXR; leukocytosis; ↑ ESR; ↑ LFTs; Biopsy showing nodular sclerosis, mixed cellularity, or lymphocytes +/− **Reed-Sternberg** cells.

Treatment: Radiation; adjuvant chemotherapy.

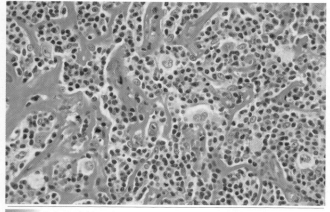

FIGURE 6.1 Hodgkin's disease/Reed-Sternberg cells. © *Barry R. DeYoung, MD, University of Iowa College of Medicine.*

History of Present Illness: A 7-year-old girl is brought to her pediatrician. Her mother is concerned because she has been having frequent **epistaxis** in school. They are not precipitated by anything, but can be severe. Physical exam shows **petechiae** and **bullae** inside her mouth.

Disease: Idiopathic Thrombocytopenic Purpura (ITP)
Pathology: Autoimmune IgG autoantibody binds to platelets → splenic Fc receptors bind antibody → platelet destruction in spleen.
Characteristics: Children and young adults; females > males; mucosal or skin bleeding; precipitated by viral infection.
Diagnosis: Clinical diagnosis; ↓ **platelets (<10,000);** prolonged bleeding time; normal PT and PTT; megathrombocytes; platelet-associated IgG.
Treatment: Splenectomy (most definitive treatment); prednisone; immunoglobulin; danazol; immunosuppressants.

♦   ♦   ♦

History of Present Illness: A 6-year-old boy presents to his pediatrician for fever and ear pain. He has fullness of his left ear and severe pain for the past 2 days. Past medical history is significant for two **otitis media** infections and four of bronchitis. He has been hospitalized for one of the **bronchitis** infections. HEENT exam reveals an infected left ear with loss of the light reflection and anatomical landmarks.

Disease: IgA Deficiency
Pathology: Defective IgA due to a genetic component, but exact etiology unknown.
Characteristics: Asymptomatic; recurrent **sinopulmonary infections** and **diarrhea.** Associated with autoimmune disorders (common variable immunodeficiency, SLE, rheumatoid arthritis).
Diagnosis: Clinical diagnosis; deficiency in IgA.
Treatment: Immunoglobulin therapy ineffective.

History of Present Illness: A 6-year-old girl is brought into her pediatrician. Her mother reports that she has been ill for the past few days. She has been noted to have some **nosebleeds** the past few days. She has had three in the past 2 days. On physical exam she appears pale and has **petechiae** on her legs. On palpation she has mild cervical **lymphadenopathy.**

Disease: Leukemia

Pathology: Malignancy of lymph or heme cells → infiltration of cells into the liver, spleen, lymph nodes, or bone marrow → differentiated by cell type and onset. Acute lymphoblastic **(ALL) (80% of acute leukemias of children);** acute myeloblastic (AML) diagnosed by presence of **Auer rods;** chronic lymphocytic (CLL); chronic myeloid leukemia (CML) due to translocation of **Philadelphia chromosome (9:22).**

Characteristics: Asymptomatic, splenomegaly, hepatomegaly, lymphadenopathy, bleeding; infection; bone pain; pallor; stomatitis or gum hypertrophy; fatigue. Children > adults in ALL and CLL. Can be induced by radiation or toxins.

Diagnosis: Clinical presentation; Coombs positive; leukocytosis; peripheral smear; Philadelphia chromosome.

Treatment: Chemotherapy; combination chemotherapy; +/− bone marrow transplant.

◆ ◆ ◆

History of Present Illness: A 62-year-old man suffers from **lower back pain.** He has noted that the pain has increased over the past month. His review is also positive for multiple respiratory **infections** this past winter. Physical exam shows mild tenderness to palpation over the sacral area. Labs ordered reveal **hypercalcemia** and an **elevated sedimentation rate.**

Disease: Multiple Myeloma

Pathology: Malignancy of plasma cells → replace normal bone marrow → anemia, bone marrow failure, infection → secretion of paraproteins → hyperviscosity syndrome, amyloid deposition in kidney.

Characteristics: Bone pain; anemia; infection; pathologic fracture; hyperviscosity syndrome; renal failure.

Diagnosis: Clinical diagnosis; hypercalcemia; normocytic normochromic anemia; RBC **rouleau** formation; elevated ESR; **Bence-Jones proteinuria** on UA; lytic lesions **"punched out"** on x-ray; monoclonal protein on immunoelectrophoresis.

Treatment: Melphalan; prednisone; chemotherapy; autologous stem-cell transplantation; radiation; bisphosphonates.

History of Present Illness: A 2-month-old baby **boy** is brought into his pediatrician because of a **white tongue.** His mom says she tries to wipe it off, but it stays white. On physical exam he has severe **diaper rash.** Also, on review of his growth chart you note that he is below the 5th percentile for his age.

Disease: Severe Combined Immunodeficiency (SCID)
Pathology: Autosomal-recessive or X-linked defect → (some due to **adenosine deaminase deficiency [ADA]**) → deficiency in **B and T cells.**
Characteristics: Severe/recurrent infections, malignancy; failure to thrive.
Diagnosis: Clinical diagnosis; adenosine deaminase deficiency; histologic findings.
Treatment: Bone marrow transplant; ADA gene transplantation.

◆   ◆   ◆

History of Present Illness: A 28-year-old **Greek** woman presents with increasing **fatigue** and **weakness.** She is otherwise healthy and does not have any significant past medical history. Her family history is significant for a grandmother with a bleeding disorder. Physical exam is within normal limits. A CBC reveals **hemoglobin of 9.0 and a hematocrit of 29.**

Disease: Thalassemia
Pathology: Hereditary defect → impaired/reduced production of alpha or beta globin chains → defective hemoglobin → hypochromic, microcytic anemia.
Characteristics: Alpha thalassemias more common in **Asians.** Beta thalassemia more common in **Mediterraneans.** Mild presentation: fatigue, weakness, pallor, splenomegaly. Moderate: growth failure, bony deformities, jaundice. Severe: hydrops fetalis in severe alpha thalassemia.
Diagnosis: ↓ hemoglobin/hematocrit; abnormal blood smear (hypochromic, target cells, **basophilic stippling** in beta thalassemia); ↓ MCV, hemoglobin electrophoresis.
Treatment: None for clinically mild; folate supplements; transfusion; splenectomy; deferoximine; allogenic bone marrow transplantation.

History of Present Illness: A 38-year-old female presents with acute onset of **visual field** defects. She says that they have been getting worse over the past 24 hours. She does not recall ever having them before. Her only other complaint is **weakness.** Her past medical history is noncontributory. On physical exam you note **petechiae** on her legs. The rest of her exam is normal.

Disease: Thrombotic Thrombocytopenic Purpura (TTP)

Pathology: Unknown etiology?? → IgG autoantibody binds to platelets → splenic sequestration of antibody-platelet complex → microangiopathic hemolytic anemia, thrombocytopenia, neurologic and renal dysfunction.

Characteristics: Fatigue; **neurologic manifestations** (HA, aphasia, altered consciousness, visual field defects); pallor; **purpura;** fever; renal insufficiency, abdominal tenderness and pain. Idiopathic commonly affects children.

Diagnosis: Anemia; reticulocytosis, abnormal smear (**schistocytes,** helmet cells, etc.); thrombocytopenia; ↑ bilirubin and LDH; UA hematuria.

Treatment: Plasmapheresis; prednisone; antiplatelet agents; splenectomy (definitive treatment).

◆　　◆　　◆

History of Present Illness: A 18-year-old female is brought into the ER of the hospital for **excessive bleeding.** She had a wisdom tooth extraction yesterday in the afternoon. She says that she has not stopped bleeding since then. On physical exam you note minimal bleeding from the gum where the tooth was located. You draw blood and find an **elevated PTT.**

Disease: von Willebrand Factor Deficiency

Pathology: Autosomal-dominant defect → defective or decreased von Willebrand factor → impaired platelet adhesion → defective coagulation.

Characteristics: Most common congenital bleeding disorder. Prolonged bleeding (mostly mucosal). Common to happen after surgery or dental procedure.

Diagnosis: ↑ PTT; ↑ bleeding time; ↓ **factor VIII;** ↓ **von Willebrand factor.**

Treatment: Supportive; desmopressin acetate; factor VIII; tranexamic acid.

HEMATOLOGY—cont'd

History of Present Illness: A 77-year-old male is seen by his nursing home physician for his annual checkup. The nurse reports that he has had **decreased interest** in participating in resident activities for the past few months. The patient states that he has had problems with his **eyes** that make it difficult to read his newspaper. On review of his history you note that he has lost **weight** over the past year. There are no gross abnormalities on physical exam.

Disease: Waldenstrom's Macroglobulinemia

Pathology: ↑ IgM-producing B cells → ↑ IgM and its paraprotein secretion → serum hyperviscosity.

Characteristics: >50 years. Present in patients with lymphoma, myeloma, and other tumors. Fatigue; lethargy; nausea; **changes in consciousness,** visual problems; **mucosal bleeds;** peripheral neuropathy; vertigo, **hepatosplenomegaly; purpura.**

Diagnosis: Anemia +/− **rouleau formation;** ↑ serum viscosity; **IgM monoclonal spike** on electrophoresis; lymphocytic infiltrate in bone marrow.

Treatment: Plasmapheresis, chemotherapy, stem-cell transplantation.

♦　　♦　　♦

History of Present Illness: A 3-year-old **male** is brought to the dermatologist for recurrent **eczema.** His past medical history is significant for hospitalization for RSV X2, pneumonia X1, and severe chicken pox. Physical exam significant for eczema covering his forearms and upper chest.

Disease: Wiskott-Aldrich Syndrome

Pathology: X-linked recessive defect on Xp11.23 → progressive loss of T lymphocytes in peripheral blood and lymph nodes → ↓ IgM, ↑ IgA and IgE.

Characteristics: Males; **thrombocytopenia; eczema;** recurrent infection; early death.

Diagnosis: Clinical diagnosis; thrombocytopenia; ↑ IgA and IgE; ↓ IgM.

Treatment: Bone marrow transplantation.

CHAPTER 7
NEUROLOGY

History of Present Illness: An 81-year-old white female presents with progressive **dysphagia** and **dysarthria** for the past 6 months. She has also been noted to have increasing gait difficulties. Patient's past medical history is significant for hyperlipidemia, hypertension, and paroxysmal atrial fibrillation. Her review of systems is significant for a 30-lb weight loss in the past few months. On physical exam she is cacectic. She has both **lower and upper extremity weakness.** Her speech is **unintelligible.** MRI of her brain is within normal limits.

Disease: Amyolotrophic Lateral Sclerosis (ALS) (AKA Lou Gehrig's Disease)

Pathology: Unknown?? Familial form related to mutation in copper-zinc dismutase gene on Chrom 21→ **upper and lower** motor-neuron deficits.

Characteristics: Dysphagia; dysarthria; respiratory difficulties; limb weakness/stiffness/wasting/spasticity; decreased deep-tendon reflexes; loss of Babinski's sign; fasciculations. **Progressive and fatal within 3–5 years.**

Diagnosis: Mildly elevated CK; **EMG**—abnormal spontaneous activity in resting muscle and decreased motor units under voluntary control. (Note: Normal CSF, head MRI/CT, TSH.)

Treatment: Riluzole; symptomatic and supportive.

NEUROLOGY—cont'd

History of Present Illness: A 76-year-old female is brought in by her daughter because she has had increasing **forgetfulness.** Her daughter says that she disoriented at times, confused, and her thoughts are **disorganized.** Her past medical history includes DM type II and a C section. She has no history of recent trauma and is not on any current medications other than glucophage. On exam she is a pleasant, cooperative, and alert woman. Screening labs (electrolytes, TSH, hemoglobin and hematocrit) are all normal.

Disease: Alzheimer's

Pathology: Unknown etiology?? May be related to the choline acetyltransferase deficiency, abnormal amyloid expression, or synaptophysin immunoreactivity → **neurofibrillary tangles, neuritic plaques, amyloid angiopathy,** and Hirano bodies found superimposed on generalized cerebral atrophy. Amount of neurofibrillary tangles corresponds with clinical impairment (Fig. 7.1).

Characteristics: Most common dementia in elderly population. **Progressive** deterioration of intellectual functioning and motor problems (can lead to paralysis). (Note: *Pick's disease presents similarly, but is more frequent in women and is characterized by Pick bodies and lobar atrophy.*)

Diagnosis: Clinical diagnosis; mental status exam; exclusion of other causes of dementia (electrolytes, calcium, glucose, TSH, B_{12}, LFT, drugs, infectious causes); CT or MRI showing diffuse atrophy.

Treatment: Donepezil; Tacrine.

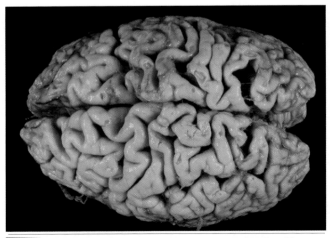

FIGURE 7.1 Alzheimer's. © *Barry R. DeYoung, MD, University of Iowa College of Medicine.*

NEUROLOGY—cont'd

History of Present Illness: A 59-year-old white female presents with recent onset weakness and **dysarthria.** Her son reports that she was sitting watching TV when she suddenly went limp and slumped over. She stayed like that for a few minutes and was disoriented when roused. Her past medical history is significant for **paroxysmal atrial fibrillation.** On physical exam she has marked weakness on her left upper and lower extremities. She also has mildly slurred speech.

Disease: Cerebrovascular Disease (Infarction, Hemorrhage, TIA)

Pathology: (1) <u>Infarction</u>—most common cause of cerebrovascular disease, caused by either thrombosis (atherosclerosis) or embolism (emboli from cardiac valves, tumor cells, fat, air). (2) <u>Hemorrhage</u>—intracerebral (due to **HTN**) or subarachnoid (AV malformations, aneurysm, trauma). (3) <u>Transient ischemic attacks</u>—rapid, transient changes in cerebral blood flow (Fig. 7.2).

Characteristics: Changes in consciousness; vomiting; headache; malaise; nausea; focal or diffuse neurologic deficits; papillary defects; ataxia. Subarachnoid hemorrhage **"worst headache of my life"** followed by nausea, vomiting, meningeal signs.

Diagnosis: Clinical diagnosis; CT/MRI.

Treatment: Dependent on the cause. (1) Infarction—anticoagulation; corticosteroids; calcium channel blockers. (2) Hemorrhage—surgical evacuation; supportive. (3) TIA—Antiplatelets, carotid endarterectomy.

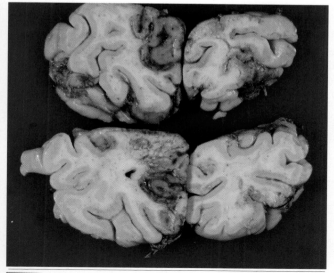

FIGURE 7.2 Cerebrovascular disease/infarction. © *Barry R. DeYoung, MD, University of Iowa College of Medicine.*

NEURO

NEUROLOGY—cont'd

History of Present Illness: A 39-year-old male is brought into the ER after a **seizure.** He is reported to have fallen down from a standing position and then to have had what sounds like a tonic-clonic seizure. His past medical history is only significant for high blood pressure. After recovering from his seizure, his review of systems reveals recent **headaches, nausea,** and malaise.

Disease: Glioblastoma Multiforme (Astrocytoma Grade IV)

Pathology: Alteration of **p53,** amplification of epidermal growth factor receptor gene (EGFR), or no discernable genetic alteration → overproliferation of glial cells.

Characteristics: Most common primary brain neoplasm. Headache, nausea, vomiting, malaise, personality changes, intellectual impairment, seizures.

Diagnosis: CT/MRI; biopsy, electroencephalogram.

Treatment: Surgical resection +/− radiation therapy.

◆   ◆   ◆

History of Present Illness: A 31-year-old male presents with bilateral lower extremity **muscle weakness** for the past week and a half. He says it is worse in his lower extremities, but seems to be **ascending.** His past medical history is significant for the "flu" with diarrhea a couple of weeks ago. On physical exam it is noted that his lower extremities have 4/5 strength and **diminished deep-tendon reflexes.**

Disease: Guillain-Barré Syndrome

Pathology: Etiology unknown?? → acute ascending polyneuropathy.

Characteristics: Symmetrical **ascending proximal muscle weakness;** flaccidity; diminished deep-tendon reflexes. Recent history of **infectious illness,** inoculation, or surgical procedures. Associated with *Campylobacter jejuni.*

Diagnosis: Clinical presentation; ↑ gamma globulin; ↓ EMG conduction; LP with ↑ protein.

Treatment: Plasmapheresis; IV immunoglobulin; supportive care (respiratory).

NEUROLOGY—cont'd

TABLE 7.1

Type	Who?	Where?	Characteristics
Glioblastoma multiforme (Astro IV)	Elderly	Cerebral	Most common primary neoplasm, malignant, **fast growing, pseudopalisading**
Metastatic tumors	Varies	Cerebral	Secondary to lung, breast, skin, GI CA
Meningioma	Women>Men, middle-late life	Cerebral	**Benign,** second most common primary neoplasm, resectable, **psammoma bodies**
Acoustic neuroma	More often in children	Cerebral hemispheres	Amplification of **N-myc** oncogene
Oligodendroglioma	Adults	Cerebral	Calcification **("fried egg cells"),** resectable
Medulloblastoma	Children	Roof of fourth ventricle effecting brainstem and **cerebellum**	Malignant, **most common tumor in children,** resectable +/− radiation or chemotherapy
Ependymoma	Children and adolescents	Ependyma of ventricle	Can **increase intracranial pressure,** resectable, not radiosensitive, **perivascular pseudorosettes.**
Retinoblastoma	Children	Retina	Hereditary and nonhereditary, **rb gene, Flexner and Wintersteiner rosettes.**

NEURO

NEUROLOGY—cont'd

History of Present Illness: A 47-year-old white **male** presents with complaints of **"restless"** legs and arms. He reports that he has had **progressive** worsening of the movements. The movements are not precipitated by any action or medication. His past medical history is significant for a grandfather with a movement disorder. On physical exam he is a well-developed male with no significant deficits. Neurological exam reveals reflexes and strength within normal limits. You note a slight **choreiform** movement of his right hand when testing his cerebellar function.

Disease: Huntington's Disease

Pathology: Autosomal-dominant genetic defect in the Huntington's disease gene **(4p16.3)** → **CAG trinucleotide repeat** → protein aggregation and intranuclear inclusions → unknown how, but structurally affects **basal ganglia** resulting in **decreased GABA** and acetylcholine or increased dopamine function. A common example of **genetic anticipation.**

Characteristics: Male, 40–50s; **choreiform;** writhing; dystonic posturing; akinesia; rigidity; dementia; change in affect. Increased risk for suicide. **Fatal** within 15–20 years.

Diagnosis: Clinical diagnosis; Huntington's disease gene.

Treatment: Phenothiazines; haloperidol; tetrabenazine; reserpine.

◆   ◆   ◆

History of Present Illness: 34-year-old white female presents with mild **weakness** and **tingling** of her left foot. She notes that it comes and goes for a few days at a time. She has noticed also that it gets worse when she steps into a hot bath or shower. On physical exam is noted that she has **relative afferent papillary defect** on the right eye. During the examination she mentions that she has recently been having pain in that eye.

Disease: Multiple Sclerosis

Pathology: Etiology unknown?? Theories point to environmental causes, genetic susceptibility, and autoimmune factors. More common in western Europeans in **temperate areas.**

Characteristics: Most common demyelinating disorder. Unilateral optic neuritis; ataxia; nystagmus; internuclear ophthalmoplegia; spasticity; incontinence.

Diagnosis: Clinical diagnosis/presentation; MRI or CT abnormalities in the periventricular or **corpus callosum;** CSF lymphocytosis, ↑ IgG **(oligoclonal bands).**

Treatment: Corticosteroids; ACTH; azathioprine; cyclophosphamide; beta interferon.

NEUROLOGY—cont'd

History of Present Illness: A 30-year-old woman presents with increasing lower limb **weakness** for the past 2 months. She notes that she does not seem to have the same energy to do things later in the day. On physical exam you note that she has some slight **ptosis** of her right eye. When examining her extraocular movements she mentions mild **diplopia.**

Disease: Myasthenia Gravis

Pathology: Autoimmune disorder caused by autoantibodies against the **acetylcholine** receptors at the neuromuscular junction → decreased **motor-neuron** action.

Characteristics: Women > men. Muscle weakness (extraocular, facial, extremities), limb weakness (**proximal** > distal); **ptosis,** diplopia, dysphagia, respiratory difficulties, **thymoma (20%).** Symptoms can fluctuate with time of day **(worse at night or following exertion).** Associated with rheumatoid arthritis and lupus.

Diagnosis: Edrophonium test (tensilon test); neostigmine test; EMG; ↑ acetylcholine receptor antibodies; CT/x-ray to look for coexisting thymoma.

Treatment: Anticholinesterase drugs; thymectomy; corticosteroids; plasmapheresis; IV immunoglobulin.

◆   ◆   ◆

History of Present Illness: A 58-year-old male complains of increasing stiffness in his joints. His wife mentions that he has also had a mild **tremor** in his left hand. This has been getting progressively worse over the past year. Past medical history is noncontributory. During the interview it is noted that he has a **flat** affect. On physical exam it is noted that, although his strength is 5/5 on upper and lower extremities, there is a **cogwheel rigidity** to his arm motions. He also has a shuffling gait.

Disease: Parkinson's Disease

Pathology: (1) Idiopathic — Etiology unknown?? → decreased dopamine in the **nigrostriatal** system. (2) Recreational **MPTP** (1- methyl-4-phenyl-1,2,5,6-tetrahydropyridine) use. (3) Injury to substantia nigra. → **depigmented substantia nigra** and **Lewy bodies.**

Characteristics: Tremor (**4–6 cycles** per second at rest), rigidity (**"cogwheel rigidity"),** bradykinesia; masklike facies; drooling; shuffling gait with decreased arm movement.

Diagnosis: Clinical diagnosis; rule out other causes of clinical presentation.

Treatment: Amantadine; anticholinergic medications (reduce tremor and rigidity); levodopa; carbidopa; dopamine agonists (bromocriptine, pergolide, pramipexole, ropinirole); selegiline; clozapine; tolcapone; thalamotomy or pallidotomy; deep brain stimulation of thalamus.

NEURO

CHAPTER 8
RENAL

History of Present Illness: A 35-year-old white male presents to the ER complaining of nausea, vomiting, and malaise for the past 24 hours. He has a history of recurrent pseudomonal infections secondary to cystic fibrosis. He is currently on day 5 of piperacillin and **gentamycin.** On laboratory examination he has hematuria, **granular casts,** and epithelial cells in his UA and an elevated BUN/creatinine ratio.

Disease: Acute Tubular Necrosis (ATN)

Pathology: Destruction of tubular epithelial cells via (1) nephrotoxicity (contrast, aminoglycosides, metals); (2) ischemia; (3) obstruction (tumors, prostatic hypertrophy, vasculitis); (4) disease (DIC, glomerulonephritis, hemolytic uremic syndrome).

Characteristics: Nausea; vomiting; malaise; changes in mental status; diffuse abdominal pain; seizures.

Diagnosis: Clinical diagnosis; FE Na $>1\%$; UA—pigmented granular casts with epithelial cells; $\uparrow$ BUN/creatinine.

Treatment: Restriction of sodium, potassium, and water intake; loop diuretics, restriction of dietary protein; nutritional support/supplementation.

RENAL—cont'd

History of Present Illness: A 3-year-old male infant is brought to you because his mother reports that she has noticed that his diapers are pink. His mom is worried because she has **chronic renal failure** herself. You examine the patient and he appears to be a healthy, well-nourished child within the 50th percentile for height and weight. His mom mentions that she has noticed that the baby is not as attentive and does not startle to loud sounds and seems inattentive when spoken to.

Disease: Alport's Syndrome
Pathology: Autosomal-dominant, autosomal-recessive, and X-linked inheritance → collagen IV defect → glomerular basement-membrane leakage → nephritic syndrome with large foam cells.
Characteristics: Hematuria; sensorineural deafness; lens dislocation; posterior cataracts; corneal dystrophy.
Diagnosis: Clinical diagnosis; biopsy showing glomerular sclerosis; **anemia;** UA—proteinuria, hematuria, RBC casts.
Treatment: ACE inhibitors; renal transplantation.

◆　　　◆　　　◆

History of Present Illness: A 50-year-old, obese, white male with a 7-year history of **hypertension** and diabetes comes into the office complaining of increased swelling in his feet. You examine his legs, and he has 2+ pitting **edema** of his legs bilaterally. He also mentions that he has an ingrown toenail that has not healed in the past 4 months. On inspection you notice an ingrown toenail with erythema and breakdown of the skin. Pedal pulses are barely palpable. PE shows a BP of 158/99. A UA shows **protein,** glucose, and **fatty casts.**

Disease: Diabetic Nephropathy
Pathology: Microangiopathy → (1) nephrotic syndrome; (2) arteriolar sclerosis; (3) chronic renal failure. See Diabetes Mellitus.
Characteristics: Most common cause of end-stage renal disease. History of diabetes. Edema of lower extremities; dyspnea; ascites; any symptoms associated with diabetes mellitus.
Diagnosis: Clinical diagnosis; fasting blood sugar/Hg A1c; ↑ BUN/ Creatinine; hypercholesterolemia; UA with blood, glucose, and protein; biopsy showing capillary BM thickening; diffuse glomerulosclerosis, nodular glomerulosclerosis; **Kimmelstiel-Wilson nodules.**
Treatment: ACE inhibitors (first line), better glycemic control; restriction of dietary protein, calcium channel blocker; dialysis; renal transplantation.

History of Present Illness: A 55-year-old male with **HIV** presents in the clinic complaining of hematuria. He has also noted that he has difficulties **breathing** when he exerts himself. The patient believes it is due to his recent weight gain. On physical exam you note a well-nourished but not obese patient. Exam is significant for 3+ pitting **edema** of his lower extremities. UA shows 3+ **protein.**

Disease: Focal Segmental Glomerulosclerosis

Pathology: Focal degeneration and damage to epithelial cells → segmental sclerosis → collapse of the basement membrane and hyalinosis. Primary/idiopathic (15%); secondary to other renal pathology; secondary to other diseases/disorders (HIV, heroin, sickle cell, obesity).

Characteristics: Hematuria; edema; hypertension; dyspnea.

Diagnosis: Clinical diagnosis; ↑ BUN and creatinine; IgM and C3 on immunofluorescence; fused foot processes on electron microscopy; **focal segmental sclerosis** on light microscopy.

Treatment: Prednisone; cytotoxic treatment for refractory patients.

◆   ◆   ◆

History of Present Illness: A 17-year-old male complains of his **third upper respiratory infection** this winter. He states that he has a runny nose, cough, abdominal discomfort, and occasionally blood in his urine. Physical exam is noncontributory. UA shows gross **hematuria** and red cell casts.

Disease: IgA Nephropathy/Berger's Disease

Pathology: IgA deposits in the mesangium → nephritic syndrome.

Characteristics: Most common **acute glomerulonephritis** in US; children and young adults; males > females; hematuria; edema; upper respiratory infection; flulike illness; end-stage renal failure in 5–10 years.

Diagnosis: Clinical diagnosis; hematuria; hypertension; ↑ serum IgA; mesangioproliferative glomerulonephritis on light microscopy; IgA mesangial deposits on electron microscopy.

Treatment: Prednisone; fish oil; renal transplantation.

RENAL—cont'd

History of Present Illness: A 40-year-old white female presents with malaise, fatigue, and joint pain. She says that her joints hurt when she tries to move. She came in because she just noticed a small amount of **hematuria.** On physical exam she appears to be a healthy 40 year old. She has a **butterfly-shaped rash** over her nose and cheeks that is made worse when she spends time in the sun. Her UA shows protein-uria and hematuria.

Disease: Lupus Nephropathy

Pathology: Anti-ds DNA → aggregations of antigen-antibody complexes in capillaries → systemic disease that consists of arthritis, photosensitivity, renal, neurologic, hematologic, and other associated autoimmune disorders.

Five types of renal disease:

    Type I—normal

    Type II—mesangial proliferative

    Type III—focal and segmental proliferative

    Type IV—diffuse proliferative

    Type V—membranous nephropathy

Characteristics: Females > males; African American > Caucasian; hereditary; can present with **either nephritic or nephrotic symptoms.**

Diagnosis: Clinical diagnosis: "Full house" of IgG, IgA, IgM, and C3 form **"Wire loops."**

Treatment: Corticosteroids; cyclophosphamide; cytotoxic; dialysis is supportive; renal transplant.

RENAL

RENAL—cont'd

History of Present Illness: A 26-year-old male comes in complaining of cough, sneezing, and headache for the past 4 days. Review of systems reveals that he also has had a fever and blood in his urine (hematuria). Physical examination shows slight erythema of the pharynx without any exudate. Lung, cardiac, and abdominal exam are all normal. 2+ pitting **edema** of the lower extremities is present. UA reveals **oval bodies** and protein.

Disease: Membranoproliferative Glomerulonephritis

Pathology: Changes in basement membrane with proliferation of glomerular cells and leukocyte infiltrate → thickening of the capillary walls and mesangium → **nephrotic or nephritic nephropathy.** Type I—**subendothelial** deposits of IgG and C3 (66%); type II—subepithelial **dense deposits** in the basement membrane (33%); type III—rare, both subendothelial and subepithelial deposition. All give "**Train track**" appearance due to the splitting of the basement membrane.

Characteristics: <30 years old; recent upper respiratory tract infection (type I); edema; **hematuria;** can present with either nephritic or nephrotic symptoms; develop to chronic renal failure.

Diagnosis: Clinical diagnosis (clinically significant edema); hematuria; ↑ BUN and creatinine; hypocomplementemia; UA—protein, fatty casts, and **oval bodies;** light microscopy showing **mesangial proliferation and basement-membrane thickening.**

Treatment: Steroids; antiplatelet therapy; (renal transplantation contraindicated because of high reoccurrence).

RENAL

History of Present Illness: A 56-year-old white male with a history of severe arthritis comes in for exacerbation of his arthritis. He complains of increased pain and swelling in his lower extremities. The **gold** therapy that he has been using does not seem to be helping the pain. On physical exam you find that he has a normal range of motion of his lower extremities, but he has 2–3+ pitting **edema** of his legs bilaterally. He mentions that he has been feeling fuller recently. UA shows 3+ **protein.**

Disease: Membranous Glomerulonephritis
Pathology: Chronic Ag-Ab complexes → nephrotic syndrome. Secondary to causes such as infection (hepatitis B or C, syphilis, schistosomiasis, malaria), **SLE,** mixed connective tissue disease, diabetes, tumors (lung and colon), and toxic agents (penicillamine, captopril, gold, **NSAIDs**).
Characteristics: Most common cause of primary nephrotic syndrome in adult. More common in >50 years; generalized edema; hematuria; progress to end-stage renal disease. Increased incidence of occult **neoplasms** of stomach, lung, and colon.
Diagnosis: Clinical diagnosis; hypoalbuminemia; hypercholesterolemia; thickening of glomerular capillary wall on light microscopy; **"Spike and dome"** IgG and C3 deposits in the basement membrane when stained with silver; IgG and C3 on immunofluorescence; deposits on subepithelial surface of BM on electron microscopy; UA—proteinuria, fatty casts, and oval fat bodies.
Treatment: Prednisone; cytotoxic agents.

◆　　　◆　　　◆

History of Present Illness: A **6-year-old male** comes in complaining of swelling of his legs and increasing abdominal discomfort. His past medical history is only significant for a recent reaction to a **bee sting** at school for which he did not need to be hospitalized. Physical exam reveals **ascites** and 2+ pitting edema bilaterally on the lower extremities.

Disease: Minimal Change Disease (AKA Lipoid Nephrosis)
Pathology: Visceral epithelial damage → fusion of foot processes → loss of negative charge → nephrotic syndrome (loss of protein).
Characteristics: Most **common nephrotic syndrome in children;** More common in males than females in younger patients. Associated with upper respiratory infections, tumors, Hodgkin's, immunizations, **hypersensitivity reactions** (NSAID, bee sting). Recurrent bacterial infections; predisposed to thromboembolic events; edema.
Diagnosis: Clinical diagnosis; **"fusion" of epithelial foot processes** on electron microscopy; normal to minimal mesangial proliferation on light microscopy.
Treatment: Prednisone; cyclophosphamide or clorambucil.

History of Present Illness: A 36-year-old woman presents with blood in her urine. She is currently being managed for infertility and has noticed increasing abdominal pain and tenderness. Your physical exam reveals borderline **hypertension** and flank tenderness. Suspicious of a **UTI** you order a UA. It reveals gross **RBCs** but no WBC or casts.

Disease: Polycystic Kidney Disease

Pathology: Genetics—Adult is **autosomal-dominant** defect in **chromosome 16 (ADPKD1 and 2)**; infantile is autosomal-recessive defect → hundreds of cysts in the cortex and medulla → progressive renal failure (Fig. 8.1).

Characteristics: Fatal in infants; presents as **hematuria, hypertension,** palpable mass, and renal failure in adults between 15–30 years. Associated with **berry aneurysms** of the circle of Willis, UTIs, nephrolithiasis, mitral valve prolapse, or other aortic abnormalities.

Diagnosis: Clinical diagnosis; hematuria on UA; CT showing cystic kidneys; ↑ BUN and creatinine.

Treatment: Supportive treatment of hypertension; dialysis; and renal transplantation.

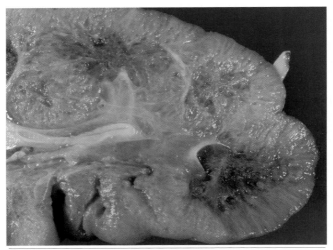

Figure 8.1 Polycystic kidney disease. © *Barry R. DeYoung, MD, University of Iowa College of Medicine.*

RENAL

RENAL—cont'd

History of Present Illness: A 10-year-old male presents to your clinic.
He complains of a slight cough and fever. His mother reports that he
suffered from a more severe **cold** last week. This past week his mother
reports that he has not been urinating as frequently. Observation
reveals a well-nourished and well-developed 10 year old. He has slight
periorbital **edema,** as well as tibial edema. UA shows RBC, **red cell
casts,** and proteinuria.

Disease: Post-Streptococcal Glomerulonephritis/Post-Infectious
Glomerulonephritis

Pathology: Infection with group A β hemolytic streptococci → granular
immune complexes → nephritis. Occasionally by Hepatitis B or C, HIV,
Staphylococcus aureus, EBV, mumps, coccidiodomycosis, toxoplasmo-
sis, or parasitic infections (malaria) in nonstreptococcal glomerulonephritis.

Characteristics: Previous infection; malaise; fever; oliguric; edema;
hypertensive.

Diagnosis: Electron microscopy displays **"humps"** of IgG, IgM, and C3 in
the mesangium and basement membrane; immunofluorescence shows
granular IgG and C3 in the mesangium and capillary basement membrane; ↓ serum complement; ↑ **Antistreptolysin O;** UA with RBC,
casts, and proteinuria **("coca-cola" or "tea-colored urine").**

Treatment: Supportive; antihypertensive medications.

◆   ◆   ◆

History of Present Illness: A 34-year-old male presents with fever,
malaise, and weight loss. A few weeks ago he had a cough and **dyspnea.** In the past he has had some **hematuria,** but recently he has had
oliguria. On physical exam he has bilateral **rales.** His UA shows red
cell casts, RBCs, and proteinuria.

Disease: Rapidly Progressive Glomerulonephritis (RPGN) (AKA Crescentic)

Pathology: Severe glomerular injury → infiltrate of parietal cells, mono-
cytes, macrophages → **crescents** → loss of renal function within
weeks to months. Type I—**Anti-GBM** (idiopathic, **Goodpasture**); type
II—immune complex-mediated disease (idiopathic, postinfectious,
SLE, Henoch-Schönlein purpura); type III—**ANCA** (associated with
vasculitides (idiopathic, **Wegener's, polyarteritis nodosa**).

Characteristics: Symptoms vary depending on the cause! Common symptoms include hematuria, hemoptysis, **oliguria,** dyspnea, purpura.

Diagnosis: ↑ BUN and creatinine; UA with RBCs, RBC casts, proteinuria;
ANCA; anti-GBM antibodies; ↑ complement; **crescents** visualized on
light microscopy; IgG, IgA, and C3 granular pattern on immunofluorescence; deposits on subepithelium; subendothelial; or mesangium.

Treatment: Supportive; antihypertensive medications; corticosteroids
and cytotoxic agents sometimes useful.

Renal.—cont'd

History of Present Illness: A 66-year-old female presents with increased **edema** in her legs. She is concerned because she feels "full" everywhere, including her tongue **(macroglossia)**. Her past medical history includes multiple myeloma. On physical exam she appears to be healthy other than 2+ pitting edema on her legs bilaterally. Her UA shows **proteinuria.**

Disease: Renal Amyloidosis

Pathology: Amyloid deposits in the mesangium and subendothelial layers → nephrotic syndrome. *Amyloid is a proteinaceous substance made up of fibril proteins (majority), P component, and other glycoproteins. Three types of amyloid proteins exist: amyloid light chain (AL), amyloid-associated (AA), and Aβ amyloid (Aβ).*

Characteristics: Proteinuria; **edema;** ascites; cardiac arrhythmias; **macroglossia;** increased risk of **multiple myeloma** and other neoplastic diseases. Progresses to end-stage renal disease in 2–3 years.

Diagnosis: CXR showing cardiomegaly; UA with proteinuria; EKG signs of restrictive cardiomyopathy; hypoproteinemia; hyperlipidemia; biopsy of organ showing **apple-green birefringence with Congo red stain.**

Treatment: Supportive; renal transplantation.

◆   ◆   ◆

History of Present Illness: A 65-year-old white male visits his family practitioner for **flank pain** for the past 24 hours. He was painting his house over the weekend, and he thinks he might have pulled a muscle. His past medical history reveals that he has a 60-pack year **smoking** history. He also complains of orange-colored urine. His UA shows gross **hematuria.**

Disease: Renal Cell Carcinoma

Pathology: Etiology is unknown?? → proximal tubule cell proliferation (clear, granular, spindle).

Characteristics: Most common renal malignancy. Weight loss; hematuria; flank pain; fever; thrombosis; ectopic production of hormones. **Smoking** is a significant risk factor. Minor risk factors include obesity, unopposed estrogen therapy, hypertension, and heavy metals.

Diagnosis: Clinical diagnosis; UA hematuria; erythrocytosis/polycythemia; anemia; hypercalcemia; CT, MRI, duplex Doppler; biopsy shows **polygonal clear cells.**

Treatment: Nephrectomy; vinblastine; interferon and IL-2 have variable response rates.

Renal—cont'd

History of Present Illness: A 65-year-old man is being given his annual physical examination. He mentions that occasionally he has **hematuria.** His social history includes working in an industrial power plant with some exposure to unknown toxins. He also has a 28-year **smoking** history. UA reveals **hematuria,** pyuria, and a few **epithelial cells.**

Disease: Transitional Cell Carcinoma (AKA Urothelial Tumor)

Pathology: Epithelial cell tumor of the bladder. Classified as papilloma, inverted papilloma, urothelial neoplasm of low malignant potential, urothelial carcinoma, carcinoma in situ (Fig. 8.2).

Characteristics: Most common bladder cancer. Males > females. Hematuria, pain/irritation with voiding, palpable masses. Increased risk if exposure to **cyclophosphamide,** phenacetin, cigarettes, and dyes.

Diagnosis: Clinical suspicion; UA with hematuria; azotemia; cytology; CT; MRI; cystoscopy; biopsy.

Treatment: Intravesical chemotherapy; transurethral resection or cystectomy; radiotherapy; combination therapy.

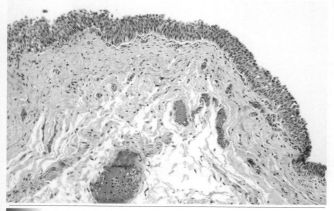

Figure 8.2 Transitional cell carcinoma. © *Barry R. DeYoung, MD, University of Iowa College of Medicine.*

History of Present Illness: A 1-year-old girl is in for her 1-year well-child care check-up. She has been healthy and growing within the 60th percentile for height and weight. On abdominal exam you notice that there is an **abdominal mass on the right side.** It is smooth, firm, and nontender.

Disease: Wilm's Tumor (Nephroblastoma)
Pathology: Genetics—WT −1 gene deletions on **Chrom 11** results in an embryonal tumor.
Characteristics: Most common malignancy of children (2–4 yrs); palpable flank mass; cryptorchidism; aniridia. **WAGR** complex (**W**ilms' tumor, **A**niridia, **G**enitourinary malformations, mental-motor **R**etardation) (Fig. 8.3).
Diagnosis: Clinical diagnosis; UA with hematuria; **urinary vanillylmandelic acid**; CT; IVP.
Treatment: Chemotherapy, radiotherapy, kidney removal.

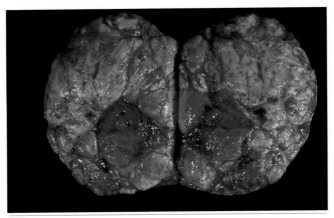

Figure 8.3 Wilm's tumor. © *Barry R. DeYoung, MD, University of Iowa College of Medicine.*

RENAL

History of Present Illness: A 50-year-old man visits the ER in the middle of the night due to severe pain in his right flank. He says that the pain has been intermittent for the past few days, but tonight it **woke him from sleep.** He says it **radiates** to his abdomen and occasionally down his right inguinal area into his testicular region. Review of systems also reveals that he is **nauseous.** Your physical exam is hard to perform because he is constantly **rolling** around.

Disease: Urolithiasis

Pathology: Calcium oxalate (CO) 80%; struvite 12%; uric acid 7%; cystine 1%.

Characteristics: Hematuria, **renal colic,** nausea, vomiting, radiating pain, urinary urgency and frequency.

Diagnosis: Clinical diagnosis; UA shows hematuria and pH <5 for uric acid or cystine stones or >7.5 if struvite stone; abdominal x-ray; renal ultrasound; CT.

Treatment: Increased fluid intake; analgesic; removal of stone; extracorporeal shock-wave lithotripsy (ESWL); decreased intake of offending agent; chelating agents.

CHAPTER 9
RESPIRATORY

History of Present Illness: A 24-year-old patient is brought into the ER status post MVA six days ago. The patient suffered from two fractured ribs and a ruptured spleen. The patient had been discharged home yesterday. This morning he woke up with a **fever.** Later on in the day he started to have difficulty breathing. On PE he is tachypnic, tachycardic, and there is a slight **retraction** of his intercostal spaces when he breathes. His CBC reveals leukocytosis. He's saturation is **68%** on 100% O_2.

Disease: Acute Respiratory Distress Syndrome (AKA Adult Respiratory Distress Syndrome)

Pathogenesis: Shock, infection (**sepsis** in one-third), aspiration, chemical injury, oxygen toxicity → diffuse alveolar capillary damage via the formation **of hyaline membranes** → pulmonary edema.

Characteristics: Hypoxia; dyspnea; tachypnea; cyanosis; heavy wet lungs.

Diagnosis: Clinical diagnosis; CXR—**"bat wing"** (parahilar) or diffuse infiltrates

Treatment: Ventilation, NO.

RESPIRATORY—cont'd

History of Present Illness: A 62-year-old Mexican man presents with increasing difficulty breathing. He just moved to the US with his son, but he worked in a **ship-building** factory in Mexico for 32 years. He normally has a **dry cough,** but would cough up blood once in while when he forgot to wear his mask during work. He was a smoker for many years, but quit 6 years ago. On P/E he has **inspiratory crackles,** clubbing, and mild cyanosis.

Disease: Asbestosis

Pathogenesis: Asbestos fibers ingested by macrophages → scarring of the lower lung fields → diffuse interstitial fibrosis (Fig. 9.1).

Characteristics: Dyspnea; **inspiratory crackles;** clubbing/cyanosis. Increased risk of **lung cancer and malignant mesotheliomas.**

Diagnosis: Clinical diagnosis; biopsy shows **ferruginous bodies;** CXR—lower lobe interstitial fibrosis; CT—pleural plaques and honeycomb appearance.

Treatment: Avoid further exposure; oral corticosteroids; pulmonary physiotherapy.

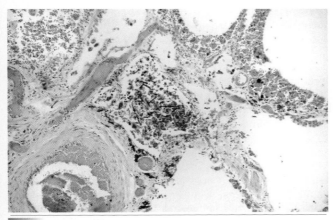

FIGURE 9.1 Asbestosis/ferruginous bodies. © *Barry R. DeYoung, MD, University of Iowa College of Medicine.*

RESPIRATORY

RESPIRATORY—cont'd

History of Present Illness: A 6-year-old girl is brought to the free health clinic because of problems breathing. The night before her mother heard her breathing really heavily and **wheezing.** She tried to rub her back to help her breath, but it did not help. Today her breathing is a better, but her mother is concerned. She is **allergic to cats,** but was not near one recently. On PE she is a healthy, alert youth in no apparent distress. Her lungs have a slight inspiratory and expiratory wheeze.

Disease: Asthma

Pathogenesis: Exposure to **antigens,** environmental chemicals/irritants, drugs, or respiratory tract infection → **inflammatory/hyperreactive airways** → thickening of the basement membrane, edema and inflammatory cell infiltrate (neutrophils, **eosinophils,** lymphocytes), hypertrophy of the submucosal glands and muscle wall → bronchoconstriction. Extrinsic—type I hypersensitivity; intrinsic—idiosyncratic.

Characteristics: Dyspnea on exertion or exposure to irritants (antigens, cold); cough; **wheezing;** complaints of chest tightness.

Diagnosis: Clinical diagnosis; decreased PFTs; peak expiratory flow meters <200 L/min; mucous plugs with **Curschmann spirals** and **Charcot-Leyden** crystals in mucus/sputum.

Treatment: Bronchodilators; corticosteroids; cromlyn; zafirkulast.

♦   ♦   ♦

History of Present Illness: A 60-year-old male miner presents to his physician for treatment of a **chronic cough.** He has no significant past medical history. His social history is significant for a 38-pack year smoking history. On physical exam you note no specific abnormalities. You order a chest x-ray, and it reveals dark **nodules** throughout his lungs but greater in the hilar regions.

Disease: Coal Worker's Pneumoconiosis/Progressive Massive Fibrosis

Pathogenesis: Inhalation of coal dust → carbon laden macrophages → **fibrosis** of the lungs and lung nodules.

Characteristics: Chronic exposure to coal; **asymptomatic;** pulmonary hypertension; cor pulmonale. **Caplan syndrome**—Rh arthritis, pheumoconiosis, and TB.

Diagnosis: Clinical diagnosis; carbon laden macrophages → linear streaks, lymph node darkening; CXR coal nodules.

Treatment: Avoid further exposure; oral corticosteroids.

RESPIRATORY—cont'd

History of Present Illness: A 61-year-old man with a **40-pack year** smoking history has been suffering from chronic **dyspnea.** It is worse when he tries to exert himself, but he is not overweight. He is seated on the edge of the examining table leaning slightly forward **breathing slowly through pursed lips.** Hemoglobin is normal and his PaO_2 is 58 mm Hg.

Disease: Emphysema

Pathogenesis: Imbalance between the proteases (elastase) and the antiproteases (due to α_1-**AT deficiency in panlobular**) → enlarged distal terminal bronchioles leading to destruction of the walls without fibrosis → ↓ elastic recoil → overinflation of the remaining airspaces and collapse on expiration → airway obstruction. Can be centrilobular, panlobular, distal acinar, or irregular emphysema (Fig. 9.2).

Characteristics: "Pink puffer"—slow forced expiration; dyspnea/dyspnea on exertion; enlarged chest cavities; **smoker.** (FYI—Smokers have an increased production of neutrophils and macrophages in their lungs → increased proteases and elastases → increased destruction of the lung.)

Diagnosis: Clinical diagnosis; CXR—bullous inflation of the lung; V/Q mismatch.

Treatment: Quit smoking; oxygen; ipratropium bromide or other sympathomimetics; oral corticosteroids.

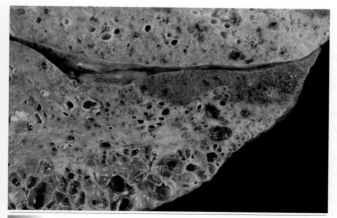

FIGURE 9.2 Emphysematous gullae. © *Barry R. DeYoung, MD, University of Iowa College of Medicine.*

RESPIRATORY

History of Present Illness: A 52-year-old man with a 50-pack year smoking history complains of a constant **productive cough** and **yellow sputum for the past 2 years.** For the past 2 days he has had an increase of the sputum production and a slight fever. He normally coughs in the morning and after that he feels better. His PaO_2 is 45 and $PaCO_2$ is 53.

Disease: Chronic Bronchitis

Pathogenesis: Chronic irritation **(smoking)** or infection → hypertrophy and hyperplasia of goblet cells → excess mucus production → obstruction of bronchioles and small bronchi.

Characteristics: "Blue bloater"; productive **cough >3 years;** mucopurulent sputum; frequent pulmonary infections; dyspnea on exertion; cyanosis; cor pulmonale (sometimes).

Diagnosis: Clinical diagnosis; CXR—increased interstitial markings **("dirty lungs")** with flattened diaphragms; hypercapnia; hypoxemia; decreased hemoglobin.

Treatment: Smoking cessation; oxygen; ipratropium bromide or sympathomimetic; theophylline; corticosteroids.

◆   ◆   ◆

History of Present Illness: A 5-year-old boy presents with cough and dyspnea on exertion. He has also had a fever for the past 3 days. His O_2 saturation is 85% on room air. On physical exam he is pale, is small for his age, and has respiratory difficulties. Past medical history significant for **recurrent upper respiratory infections.** His lungs have ronchi throughout and diminished air movement in the right lower lobe. A chest x-ray confirms a right lower lobe pneumonia. It is his **third pneumonia** this year.

Disease: Cystic Fibrosis

Pathogenesis: Autosomal-recessive mutation in **Chrom 7** (CFTR) → altered water and chloride transport of epithelial cells→ increased **viscous secretions** → organ obstruction → dilatation of glands → damage to the exocrine organ (Fig. 9.3).

Characteristics: Chronic pulmonary disease (cough, pneumonia); pancreatic insufficiency; **meconium ileus;** susceptible to *Pseudomonas aeruginosa.*

Diagnosis: Clinical diagnosis, pilocarpine iontophoresis **"sweat test";** CXR hyperinflation; hypoxemia; decreased O_2 sat.

Treatment: Prophylactic antibiotics; chest physiotherapy; cough suppressants; vaccination against pneumococcal and influenza infections; recombinant human deoxyribonuclease; lung transplantation.

RESPIRATORY—cont'd

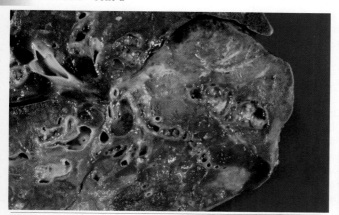

FIGURE 9.3 Cystic fibrosis. © Barry R. DeYoung, MD, University of Iowa
College of Medicine.

History of Present Illness: A 35-year-old man comes in with a 1-month
history of increased coughing. This past week he has had some
hemoptysis and difficulties breathing. He admits to smoking one
pack/day for the past 20 years. He has also noted that his urine is
orange in color. His urinary analysis shows **hematuria,** proteinuria,
and oliguria. His blood work also shows that he has **iron-deficiency
anemia.**

Disease: Goodpasture's Syndrome

Pathogenesis: Anti-basement membrane antibodies → rapidly progressive glomerulonephritis and hemorrhagic interstitial pneumonitis.

Characteristics: Hemoptysis; glomerulonephritis; men in their 20s;
cough; hypoxemia. "There are two Goodpastures—one through the
lungs (hemoptysis) and the other through the kidneys (hematuria)."

Diagnosis: Clinical diagnosis; CXR—focal pulmonary consolidation;
immunofluorescent **linear IgG;** anti-glomerular basement membrane
antibody.

Treatment: Methylprednisolone with cyclophosphamide (or other
immunosuppressant) and plasmapheresis.

RESPIRATORY—cont'd

History of Present Illness: A 67-year-old man presents with progressive **dyspnea** and has had a slight cough for the past 6 months. He **was never a smoker nor has had exposure to any toxic chemicals.** On physical exam he has mild cyanosis and mild inspiratory crepitice. A chest x-ray is ordered and it reveals a **fibrosis** of lungs alternating with areas of normal lung (honeycomb).

Disease: Idiopathic Pulmonary Fibrosis (AKA Chronic Interstitial Pneumonitis, Hamman-Rich Syndrome, Diffuse/Cryptogenic Fibrosing Alveolitis)
Pathogenesis: Chronic inflammation/injury of alveolar wall → diffuse interstitial inflammation → (edema and inflammatory cells) and fibrosis hypoxemia and cyanosis.
Characteristics: Dyspnea; cough; rapid progression with a median survival of 4 years after onset of symptoms. Present in 6th to 7th decade. **Hamman-Rich** syndrome is a familial, rapidly progressive form of the disease.
Diagnosis: Clinical diagnosis; CXR—**honeycomb lung;** CT—lung parenchymal fibrosis; biopsy shows pulmonary edema, intra-alveolar exudate, and hyaline membranes.
Treatment: Oral corticosteroid; oxygen.

◆   ◆   ◆

History of Present Illness: A 26-year-old male presents to his primary care physician for evaluation of a **cough.** His cough has been present for the past week and is productive in nature. His review of systems is negative for fever, chills, or other constitutional symptoms. Past medical history is significant for **recurrent sinusitis** as a child. On physical exam you note abnormal heart sounds. You perform an EKG and realize that he has **dextrocardia.**

Disease: Kartagener's Syndrome (AKA Immotile Cilia Syndrome)
Pathogenesis: Autosomal-recessive defect → defect in **dynein** arms → immotile cilia → impaired respiratory clearance (increased respiratory infections) and immotile spermatozoa (infertility).
Characteristics: Situs inversus; sterility; impaired respiratory defense/increased susceptibility to infections.
Diagnosis: Clinical diagnosis; normocytic, normochromic anemia; ↓ PFT; immotile sperm; CXR showing situs inversus or dextrocardia; absence of dynein arms in bronchial cilia.
Treatment: Symptomatic treatment.

RESPIRATORY—cont'd

History of Present Illness: A 75-year-old woman presents with increasing **cough** and **has had dyspnea** for the past 3 months. She has had several episodes of **hemoptysis** as well. Her review of systems is significant for a 20-lb unintentional **weight loss** over the past month and a half. She also has a **100-pack year** history. Her physical exam is significant for a cacectic woman with an inspiratory wheeze. Her lungs sounds are diminished on the right lower lobe.

Disease: Lung Cancer

Pathology: Cigarette smoking, radiation, asbestos, heavy metals, air pollution → genetic alterations in lung cells → squamous cell carcinoma (25%–40%), adenocarcinoma (25%–40%), small cell carcinoma (20%–25%), large cell carcinoma (10%–15%). **Sq**uamous and **small** cell cancer (associated with **smoking**) arise centrally, all others are peripheral. "**Small, Sq**uacking Men **Smoking** like to stand in the **CENTER** of attention" (Fig. 9.4).

Characteristics: # 1 cause of cancer. Cough; hemoptysis; wheezing; anorexia; weight loss; dyspnea; chest pain. A whole SPHERE of complications (**S**uperior vena cava syndrome; **P**ancoast's tumor; **H**orner's syndrome; **E**ndocrine (paraneoplastic); **R**ecurrent laryngeal symptoms; **E**ffusions). Metastases common to brain, bone, and liver.

Diagnosis: Chest x-ray showing masses, infiltrates; atelectasis, or pleural effusions; cytologic diagnosis (sputum, pleural effusion; **biopsy**); CT/MRI to stage or confirm diagnosis.

Treatment: Surgical resection; chemotherapy; radiation therapy.

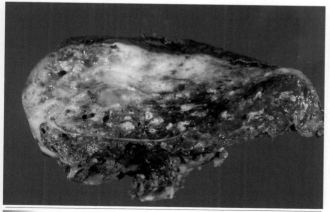

FIGURE 9.4 Lung cancer. © Barry R. DeYoung, MD, University of Iowa College of Medicine.

RESPIRATORY

History of Present Illness: A 28-year-old woman delivers at **34** weeks to a AGA baby girl. The pregnancy is complicated by **diabetes mellitus** and one previous elected abortion. The baby is delivered via **Cesarian section** due to fetal distress. The baby is **resuscitated** successfully at birth. Within the next 15 minutes the baby's breathing becomes labored and coarse. On physical exam the baby is mildly cyanotic and **has retraction of the lower ribs. Rales** are heard over both lung fields.

Disease: Neonatal Respiratory Distress Syndrome

Pathogenesis: Decreased production of type II alveolar cells → ↓ in pulmonary surfactant **(dipalmitoyl phosphatidylecholine)** → increased surface tension within the alveoli → alveoli collapse and become **atelectatic** due to decreased compliance.

Characteristics: Fine **rales;** cyanosis; difficulty **breathing** within the first 30 minutes.

Diagnosis: Clinical hypoxia of neonate; CXR with reticulogranular densities **("ground glass").**

Treatment: Replace surfactant; oxygen +/− ventilators; cortisol; insulin; prolactin; thyroxine.

◆   ◆   ◆

History of Present Illness: A 65-year-old man presents with progressive **hoarseness** of his voice. It started about 3 months ago and has gotten progressively worse. He also complains of weird sensations and sweating **(anhydrosis)** on the right side of his face. His physical exam reveals a slight **ptosis** on the right side of his face with concurrent miosis.

Disease: Pancoast's Tumor

Pathogenesis: Apical tumor impinging on the sympathetic plexus.

Characteristics: Hoarseness; miosis; **CN IX or XI** abnormalities; sympathetic abnormalities. **Horner's syndrome—anhydrosis, ptosis, miosis.**

Diagnosis: Clinical diagnosis; CXR.

Treatment: Removal of the tumor; laryngoplastic phonosurgery (to relieve vocal cord tension).

RESPIRATORY—cont'd

History of Present Illness: A 76-year-old woman has been in the hospital for the past 7 days. She was brought from the nursing home because of a hacking cough and fever for 3 days. While in the hospital she was given IV antibiotics for pneumonia. This afternoon she was found **gasping for air** and complaining of **chest pain.** She tried to get to the bathroom, but felt **dizzy** and almost fell. On physical exam she was breathing rapidly and had developed a **ventricular gallop** and a **split S_2.** An EKG shows sinus tachycardia and **nonspecific ST and T wave changes.**

Disease: Pulmonary Embolism

Pathogenesis: Embolus formation due to foreign substance (air, fat, amniotic fluid, tumor cells, or parasite eggs) or **vein thrombosis** (most often deep veins of the **leg—95%**) → occlusion of the pulmonary arteries → infarction and hemorrhage of the lungs → hypoxia → death. Can cause acute cor pulmonale. **Virchow's triad—blood stasis, endothelial damage, hypercoagulable state** (Fig. 9.5).

Characteristics: Acute **dyspnea;** chest pain/pain with inspiration; hypotension; tachypnea; cough/hemoptysis.

Diagnosis: Clinical diagnosis; **pulmonary angiography** (gold standard); EEG; V/Q scan; US/Doppler; **Homan's sign;** CXR with Hampton's hump; MRI/CT; Pathology—grossly can see large saddle emboli.

Treatment: Supportive; thrombolytic; embolectomy; anticoagulation (Heparin/or Coumadin).

RESPIRATORY

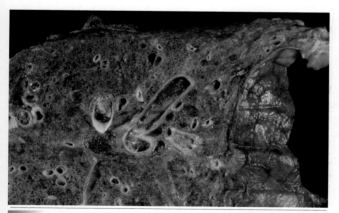

FIGURE 9.5 Pulmonary embolism. © *Barry R. DeYoung, MD, University of Iowa College of Medicine.*

RESPIRATORY—cont'd

History of Present Illness: A 37-year-old African American woman has had **tender nodules** on both of her legs for the past month. She does not recall any trauma, but has been feeling tired and achy. She has also noticed that she is **short of breath.** CBC shows **lymphopenia** and **eosinophilia.** Chest x-ray reveals **hilar lymphadenopathy.**

Disease: Sarcoidosis
Pathogenesis: ??? → **Systemic noncaseating granulomas.**
Characteristics: Women > men; **black** > white; interstitial fibrosis; fever; malaise; dyspnea; chest pain; **erythema nodosum;** splenomegaly; hepatomegaly; lymphadenopathy; skin, eyes, liver, CNS, heart, or kidney abnormalities.
Diagnosis: Clinical diagnosis; ↑ **ACE; hypercalcemia/hypercalciuria;** gammaglobulinemia; ↑ ESR; leukopenia; CXR—**bilateral hilar lymphadenopathy; Biopsy showing noncaseating granulomas.**
Treatment: Oral corticosteroids.

◆   ◆   ◆

History of Present Illness: A 65-year-old man comes in with progressive **dyspnea on exertion.** He also mentions that he has a dry **cough** that does not seem to go away. He is not a smoker, but mentions that his wife is. He has worked at a **quarry** for the past 30 years. Auscultation of his chest reveals **dry inspiratory crackles.** Chest x-ray reveals **calcified hilar lymph nodes.**

Disease: Silicosis
Pathogenesis: Inhaled silicon dioxide (silica) → macrophages ingest silica → activation of cell mediators via interaction with epithelial cells → injury and fibrosis of the lungs and the production of silicotic nodules.
Characteristics: Most common occupational disease in the world; chronic exposure; silicotuberculosis when concurrent with TB.
Diagnosis: Clinical diagnosis; CXR—**"eggshell" calcifications of hilar lymph nodes, apical blackened nodules;** biopsy of nodules shows silica under polarized light.
Treatment: Avoid further exposure; oral corticosteroids.

RESPIRATORY—cont'd

History of Present Illness: A 57-year-old man who suffers from **chronic sinusitis.** He presents to the clinic for a severe sinus infection. For the past few weeks he has been feeling tired, and he aches all over and has been losing weight. He started noticing **blood** in the tissues when he blows his nose. PE reveals bulging tympanic membranes and **multiple ulcers** in his nose.

Disease: Wegener's Granulomatosis

Pathogenesis: Autoimmune or hypersensitivity reaction → **(1) acute necrotizing granulomas of the upper respiratory tract; (2) focal necrotizing/granulomatous vasculitis of the small to medium sized vessels; (3) renal granulomas** (Fig. 9.6).

Characteristics: Pneumonitis; mucosal granulomas and ulcerations in the nose, palate, and pharynx; arthralgias; skin rash; weight loss; renal disease.

Diagnosis: Clinical diagnosis; **c-ANCA (approximately 90%),** CXR— multiple nodular infiltrates; biopsy with necrotizing granulomas in upper and lower respiratory tract; anemia; leukocytosis; throbocytosis; elevated ESR.

Treatment: Corticosteroids and cyclophosphamide.

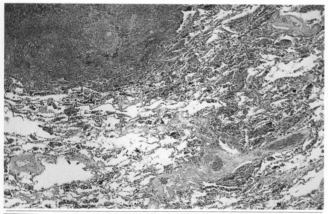

FIGURE 9.6 Wegener's granulomatosis. © *Barry R. DeYoung, MD, University of Iowa College of Medicine.*

RESPIRATORY

CHAPTER 10
RHEUMATOLOGY

History of Present Illness: A woman gives birth at 38 weeks' gestation to a healthy baby boy. At his 6-month well-child checkup the mother mentions that she has noticed that the baby is not built proportionate. He has long arms and legs compared to his torso. He appears to be reaching his developmental milestones. On physical exam you note that he is **below the 5th** percentile in growth.

Disease: Achondroplasia (most common cause of dwarfism)
Pathology: Autosomal-dominant genetic mutation in the gene for FGF receptor 3 → overproliferation of cartilage → epiphyseal plates seal off.
Characteristics: Shortened proximal extremities; normal trunk; large frontal boss; depressed nasal bridge; *no change in longevity, intelligence, or reproductive capabilities.*
Diagnosis: Clinical diagnosis; abnormal growth plates on x-ray.
Treatment: None.

♦   ♦   ♦

History of Present Illness: A 20-year-old male complains of increasing **back pain** that radiates down his thighs. He feels like his joints are very stiff, especially his hip. On physical exam his strength is 5/5 on all four extremities. He has point tenderness over his sacroiliac joints. There is an erythematous region of skin over his eyelids **(heliotrope rash).**

Disease: Ankylosing Spondylitis (AKA Marie-Strümpell Disease)
Pathology: ?? Theories include viral infection, genetic causes, or autoimmune causes → chronic inflammatory disease → increasing stiffness and pain in axial skeleton
Characteristics: Males > females; muscle weakness; muscle tenderness; **arthritis;** stooped posture; uveitis; rash **(Gottron's sign** on dorsum of hand; heliotrope over the eyelids). Also associated with lung fibrosis, **aortic arch insufficiency,** and cauda equina syndrome.
Diagnosis: Clinical diagnosis; ↑ ESR; myoglobinuria; muscle biopsy; **HLA-B27;** x-ray **"bamboo spine"** (fused spine).
Treatment: Exercise/PT; corticosteroids; NSAIDs.

RHEUMATOLOGY—cont'd

History of Present Illness: A 42-year-old male presents with a painful hip. He does not recall any recent trauma. He states that it has been getting increasingly painful over the past 2 months. He also has been feeling mild malaise. On physical exam you note a palpable painful nodule on his right hip.

Disease: Chondrosarcoma

Pathology: Malignant cartilage tumor. Categorized based on site: intramedullary vs juxtacortical. Also organized by cell type: clear cell, hyaline, myxoid (conventional), undifferentiated, and mesenchymal.

Characteristics: Males > females; presents around 4th to 5th generation; bone pain greater in the axial skeleton (pelvis, shoulder, ribs); pathologic fractures; preexisting enchondroma. Good prognosis.

Diagnosis: X-ray; biopsy.

Treatment: Surgical excision $+/-$ chemotherapy.

◆   ◆   ◆

History of Present Illness: A **3-year-old boy** comes in for his annual physical exam. His mother notes that he has been getting increasingly **clumsy.** She says that it appears as if he is regressing on some of his physical milestones. You note that as he gets onto the exam table, he uses his arms to pull himself up instead of his legs. Physical exam reveals mild hypertrophy of his calves.

Disease: Duchenne's Muscular Dystrophy

Pathology: X-linked recessive genetic defect on **Xp21** or a random mutation that codes for **dystrophin** $\rightarrow$ abnormal/decreased dystrophin $\rightarrow$ degeneration and necrosis of muscle fibers.

Characteristics: 1/10,000 males; progressive muscle weakness and muscle wasting **(pelvic, shoulder girdle);** cognitive impairment; pseudohypertrophy; heart failure; eventually death due to respiratory or cardiac failure.

Diagnosis: Clinical diagnosis; $\uparrow$ serum kinase; **EMG;** prenatal DNA testing.

Treatment: Supportive; PT; orthopedic procedures.

History of Present Illness: A 21-year-old boy presents to his physician with increased shortness of breath and fatigue. His past medical history is significant for a fracture of his left leg. Following the fracture he required surgical repair of several vessels. Physical exam reveals a healthy, appropriately developed male with a **pulsating, palpable mass** in his abdomen.

Disease: Ehlers-Danlos

Pathology: Defect in **collagen** synthesis → ten varieties with different degrees of severity and clinical presentations. Type VI is the most common autosomal-recessive form.

Characteristics: Hyperextensible skin and joints; increased elasticity of internal structures (i.e., **aortic aneurysm, ruptured colon**); retinal detachment; ruptured cornea.

Diagnosis: Clinical diagnosis; angiogram showing multiple aortic dilations; barium studies.

Treatment: Supportive; decrease risk of injury/fractures; surveillance for vascular or musculoskeletal abnormalities; surgical repair.

◆　　◆　　◆

History of Present Illness: A **12-year-old boy** comes into the ER after a soccer game. He has had increasing pain and swelling of his right femur for the past few months. Today, during the game he collided with another classmate of his. He heard a loud popping noise and has been in pain ever since. X-ray shows a fracture of his **distal femur.** The x-ray shows a "moth eaten" appearance of the fracture. The only margins visible are covered with a thin layer of new bone creating an **onion skin** appearance.

Disease: Ewing's Sarcoma

Pathology: t (11:22) (approximately 85%); t (21:21); t (7:22) → malignant tumor of **small, round cells** in bone.

Characteristics: Boys > girls; 10–15 years old at presentation; Caucasian > African American; diathesis of long bones; painful enlarging mass; swelling around site; fever.

Diagnosis: Clinical diagnosis; x-ray showing **onion-skinning** of new reactive bone; CT; MRI; ↑ ESR; ↑ WBC; anemia.

Treatment: Chemotherapy; surgery; radiation.

RHEUMATOLOGY—cont'd

History of Present Illness: A 26-year-old woman complains of increasing pain in her left shin when she runs each morning. She has no significant past medical history and was previously healthy. She does not recall any trauma to the area. Physical exam findings include a **mass** palpated on the medial surface of her knee. An x-ray reveals a large mass with a **"soap-bubble"** appearance on her femoral condyle.

Disease: Giant Cell Tumor
Pathology: Benign tumor of the osteoclasts called giant cells (Fig. 10.1).
Characteristics: Mets to lung; pain at joint (epiphyseal end of long bones (especially **femur and tibia**); pathologic fracture.
Diagnosis: X-ray; CT; MRI—can show lytic or **"soap-bubble"** appearance.
Treatment: Surgery.

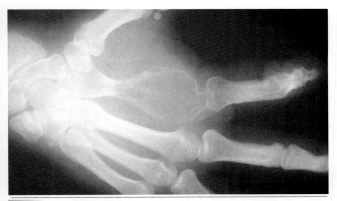

FIGURE 10.1 Giant cell tumor. © *Barry R. DeYoung, MD, University of Iowa College of Medicine.*

RHEUMATOLOGY

RHEUMATOLOGY—cont'd

History of Present Illness: A 57-year-old male presents with increasing pain in his left foot. He states that he has noticed intermittent pain in his left **midfoot.** He reports that it gets worse after drinking a few **beers** on the weekend. You note that his left foot is slightly swollen and tender around the area. You aspirate the fluid in his foot and note **needle-shaped** crystals of sodium urate that are **negatively birefringent crystals** (green) when viewed under compensated polariscopic examination.

Disease: Gout

Pathology: Increased uric acid due to ↓ excretion/ ↑ production, Lesch-Nyhan, PRPP excess, or glu-6-phosphatase deficiency → deposition of **monosodium urate** crystals at joints → phagocytosis of crystals → inflammation of joints (Fig. 10.2). *Pseudogout is deposition of calcium pyrophosphate crystal in large joints to produce basophilic rhomboid crystals. No treatment available.*

Characteristics: Male > females; genetic predisposition; **podagra** (great toe nodule); renal failure; tophi on ears, hands, feet, Achilles tendon. Pain precipitated by alcohol or fatty meals.

Diagnosis: Clinical diagnosis; ↑ serum uric acid; **needle-shaped, negatively birefringent** crystals under polarized light; renal disease; later in disease **"rat bite"** lesions in cortical bone.

Treatment: Colchicine; NSAID; Allopurinol; Probenecid; remove/decrease stimulating factors.

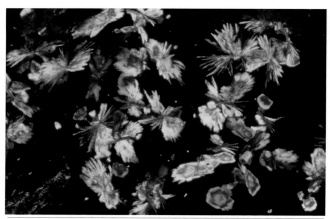

FIGURE 10.2 Gout crystals. © *Barry R. DeYoung, MD, University of Iowa College of Medicine.*

RHEUMATOLOGY—cont'd

History of Present Illness: A **16-year-old male** presents for his annual sports physical. His only complaint is changes in his vision. He states that he has had increased difficulties seeing things far away **(myopia)**. Physical is only significant for a thin youth with exceptionally **long arms and fingers.**

Disease: Marfan's Syndrome

Pathology: Autosomal genetic defect with the fibrillin gene on **chromosome 15** → defects in **elastin** → abnormalities of the skeletal system, ocular system, and cardiovascular system.

Characteristics: Males > females; tall; **long legs and arms; ectopic lentis; aortic dilation** or dissection; **mitral valve prolapse;** aortic valve insufficiency.

Diagnosis: Clinical diagnosis; genetic defect on chromosome 15.

Treatment: Regular checkup with ophthalmology and orthopedics; annual echocardiograms; endocarditis prophylaxis; prophylactic aortic root replacement.

◆   ◆   ◆

History of Present Illness: A 55-year-old man presents with a fracture of his left **distal radius.** He was playing softball this afternoon and was accidentally stepped on by the baseman as he slid into first. He has had some noted pain in that arm for the past 4 months that he attributes to "old age." The x-ray of his arm shows a complete fracture through a **cystic** lesion at the distal end of the left radius.

Disease: Osteitis Fibrosa Cystica/von Recklinghausen's

Pathology: Primary or secondary hyperparathyroidism → increased osteoclast activity → excessive bone reabsorption → cystic degeneration/**brown cystic tumors.**

Characteristics: Women > men; **hypercalcemia;** bone pain; pathologic fractures; renal stones; polyuria/polydipsia; nephrogenic diabetes insipidus; depression; psychosis; renal failure. *(Any clinical finding with hypercalcemia)* **"bones, stones, abdominal groans, and psychiatric overtones."**

Diagnosis: Hypercalcemia; hypophosphatemia; hypercalcemia; ↑ alkaline phosphatase; ↑ uric acid in serum; ↑ chloride in serum; parathyroid adenoma on US, CT, or MRI.

Treatment: Parathyroidectomy; bisphosphonates; increased fluids; estrogen replacement therapy; calcium acetate; calcitriol.

History of Present Illness: A 58-year-old woman presents with increasing pain in her knees. She has mild **swelling** in her fingers. On further questioning she states that her pain is **relieved by rest** and is **not associated with morning stiffness.** Musculoskeletal exam reveals normal reflexes and strength globally. Her knees have limited range of motion bilaterally. Also, you note some swelling in her right 3rd and 4th **DIP joints.**

Disease: Osteoarthritis
Pathology: Articular cartilage degeneration +/− overproliferation of bone **(osteophytes).**
Characteristics: More common in advanced ages; pain; loss of range of motion; cervical or lumbar pain; osteophytes at **DIP (Heberden's nodes).**
Diagnosis: Clinical diagnosis; x-ray showing osteophytes, loss of articular joint space, subchondial cysts.
Treatment: Weight loss; physical therapy; acetaminophen; triamcinolone injection; joint replacement.

♦   ♦   ♦

History of Present Illness: A 28-year-old male presents with pain in his left upper tibia. He has noted a painful nodule at this area. He has no other complaints. His physical exam is unremarkable, except for this mass at his hip.

Disease: Osteochondroma **(most common benign tumor)**
Pathology: Benign bone tumor.
Characteristics: Males > females; young; lower end of **femur** or upper tibia; pain or swelling; palpable enlargements; pathologic fractures.
Diagnosis: X-ray; CT; MRI; biopsy.
Treatment: Surgical excision.

RHEUMATOLOGY—cont'd

History of Present Illness: A 15-year-old boy comes in cradling his right arm. He states that he tripped and fell in school. Past medical history is significant for **three previous fractures.** Physical exam reveals a healthy adolescent with **blue sclera.** An x-ray shows a distal fracture of his radius.

Disease: Osteogenesis Imperfecta
Pathology: Genetic defect on **chromosome 7 or 17** → deficiency in **type 1** collagen → multiple skeletal abnormalities.
Characteristics: Four types of OI with various manifestations. Some of the presentations include **multiple fractures caused by minimal trauma; blue sclera;** ligamentous laxity; short stature; mitral valve prolapse; **hearing loss;** dental abnormalities; can be incompatible with life.
Diagnosis: Clinical diagnosis; x-ray.
Treatment: Supportive; prevention of fractures.

◆   ◆   ◆

History of Present Illness: A 54-year-old African American male presents with increasing pain in his left arm. His past medical history is positive for **intravenous drug** use. For the past few weeks he has had intermittent chills and **fevers.** A blood culture grows out **Pseudomonas.**

Disease: Osteomyelitis
Pathology: Inflammation of bone and marrow due to infection (bacterial, viral, fungal, and parasitic) (Fig. 10.3).
Characteristics: *Staphylococcus aureus* (90%); pain; fever; malaise; chills. **Salmonella** associated with **sickle cell** and **Pseudomonas** with **IV drug** users. Tuberculosis osteomyelitis presents similarly.
Diagnosis: X-ray; MRI; biopsy and culture; leukocytosis; blood culture.
Treatment: Appropriate antibiotics +/− surgical debridement/drainage.

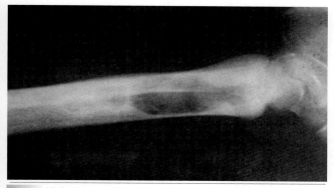

FIGURE 10.3 Osteomyelitis. © *Barry R. DeYoung, MD, University of Iowa College of Medicine.*

RHEUMATOLOGY

Rheumatology—cont'd

History of Present Illness: A 12-year-old boy presents to the ER for a presumed fracture of his left index finger. The boy had been playing basketball when he heard a cracking sound. His past medical history is significant for **three other fractures** in the past 4 years. X-rays reveal a broken index finger. The rest of his physical exam shows a healthy, well-developed, age-appropriate boy.

Disease: Osteopetrosis
Pathology: Hereditary osteoclast dysfunction → skeletal sclerosis. One variant associated with carbonic anhydrase II deficiency.
Characteristics: Multiple fractures; anemia; hydrocephaly; splenomegaly (due to extramedullary hematopoiesis); cranial nerve problems.
Diagnosis: Clinical diagnosis; x-rays.
Treatment: Bone marrow transplant.

◆　　◆　　◆

History of Present Illness: A 52-year-old woman visits her family physician for her annual checkup. Her review of systems is only significant for back pain and a noted decrease in her height. Her physical exam reveals a healthy **postmenopausal** woman with no physical abnormalities. Her physician suggests a DEXA scan of her bones.

Disease: Osteoporosis
Pathology: ↑ absorption and/or ↓ synthesis of bone → ↓ bone mass.
Characteristics: Most common hereditary bone disease. Hereditary; **fractures; loss of height;** lumbar lordosis or kyphoscoliosis.
Diagnosis: X-ray/CT/MRI showing demineralization of the spine and pelvis or compression of the vertebrae; DEXA scan showing decreased bone density.
Treatment: Increase physical activity; diet (calcium and vitamin D); estrogen; bisphosphonates.

◆　　◆　　◆

History of Present Illness: A 14-year-old boy presents in the ER following a fight with his brother. He is complaining that his left leg has been hurting and that, after being kicked by his brother, it hurts even more. Physical exam reveals a tender leg with minimal swelling and redness. An x-ray shows a break of his tibia suggestive of a **pathologic fracture.**

Disease: Osteosarcoma
Pathology: Deletion in chromosome 13 or translocation → malignant bone tumor.
Characteristics: Most common bone tumor in children. Pain; swelling; **pathologic fractures.**
Diagnosis: X-ray; biopsy.
Treatment: Surgical resection and chemotherapy.

RHEUMATOLOGY—cont'd

History of Present Illness: A 50-year-old female presents with **pain** in her legs. She has no significant past medical history or recent trauma involving her legs. Review of systems is positive for **headaches.** Her physical exam is essentially normal, except for a slight **bowing** of her legs.

Disease: Paget's Disease (AKA Osteitis Deformans)

Pathology: Cyclic disorder of osteoblastic activity → osteoclastic activity → abnormal bone mass. Evidence points to a possible association with *paramyxovirus* (Fig. 10.4).

Characteristics: Asymptomatic; bone **pain;** kyphosis; bowed tibias; **deaf;** headaches; pathologic fractures; *leontiasis ossea* (overgrowth of craniofacial skeleton); AV shunts; osteoarthritis secondary to bony malformations.

Diagnosis: X-ray; ↑ **alkaline phosphatase;** ↑ urine hydroxyproline; serum calcium can be elevated.

Treatment: Bisphosphonates; calcitonin.

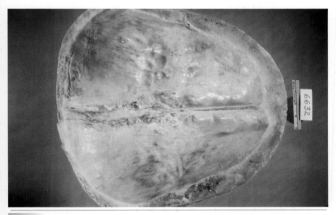

FIGURE 10.4 Paget's disease. © *Barry R. DeYoung, MD, University of Iowa College of Medicine.*

RHEUMATOLOGY

History of Present Illness: A 40-year-old woman with a history of **psoriasis** presents with increasing pain in the fingers in her left hand (arthritis). She also mentions that her lower back hurts. On physical exam you note that the fingers on her left hand are swollen and the joints are barely palpable. She also has point tenderness in at the **sacroiliac joint.**

Disease: Psoriatic Arthritis
Pathology: Inflammatory
Characteristics: Psoriasis; arthritis (asymmetric most often); inflammation of tendon sheaths **(sausage fingers)**; conjunctivitis; iritis.
Diagnosis: Clinical diagnosis; x-ray showing **pencil-in-cup** deformities, syndesmophytes, or **sacroiliitis.**
Treatment: NSAIDs; corticosteroids; antimalarial; gold; methotrexate.

RHEUMATOLOGY—cont'd

History of Present Illness: A 36-year-old woman presents with increasing pain in her hands **bilaterally.** She started noticing pain in them about 2 years ago, but they have been getting progressively worse. **She also complains of morning stiffness.** While she is speaking you notice **flexion of the DIP and extension of the PIP joints** on her right hand. On physical exam her joints are swollen and tender. The rest of her exam is normal.

Disease: Rheumatoid Arthritis

Pathology: Autoimmune systemic inflammation of synovial membranes, associated with **HLA-DR4** → pannus formation → arthritis (Fig. 10.5).

Characteristics: Females > males; **symmetrical** pain and stiffness of joints; **worse in the AM;** rheumatoid nodules; malaise; weight loss; fever.

Diagnosis: Clinical diagnosis; **rheumatoid factor;** x-ray showing **pannus** formation, erosion, osteoporosis; ↑ ESR; ↑ WBC; ↑ platelets.

Treatment: Weight loss; exercise; NSAIDs; methotrexate; antimalarial; gold; corticosteroids; assistive devices (cane, walker); splints; joint replacement.

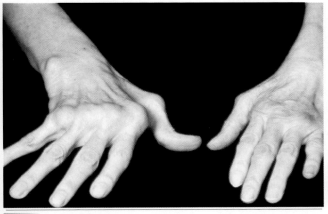

FIGURE 10.5 Rheumatoid arthritis. © *Barry R. DeYoung, MD, University of Iowa College of Medicine.*

RHEUMATOLOGY

History of Present Illness: A 37-year-old African American female presents to her family care physician with **fatigue** and **joint pain.** Her review of systems is only significant for those complaints. Her past medical history reveals empiric treatment for **tuberculosis** due to a positive PPD. She does not remember the names of the exact medications that she is taking. Her physical exam reveals only a slight **rash on cheeks and nose.**

Disease: Systemic Lupus Erythematosus (SLE)

Pathology: Anti-ds DNA → aggregations of antigen-antibody complexes → increase in inflammatory cells and mediators. Medications (procainamide, INH, phenytoin, hydralazine) (Fig. 10.6).

Characteristics: Fever; fatigue; weight loss; joint pain; **malar rash;** pleuritis; pericarditis; nonbacterial verrucous endocarditis **(Libman-Sacks endocarditis);** Raynaud's; SLE **nephrotic syndrome** (see Renal under Lupus Nephropathy). Recent medication change.

Diagnosis: Clinical diagnosis; **ANA** (sensitive); **double-stranded DNA** (anti-ds DNA) (specific to SLE); **anti-Smith antibodies** (anti-Sm) (specific to SLE). Can produce a false-positive RPR/VDRL.

Treatment: Corticosteroids.

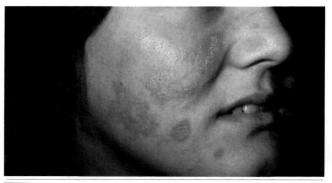

FIGURE 10.6 Systemic lupus erythematosus. © *Mary Stone, MD, University of Iowa College of Medicine.*

INDEX

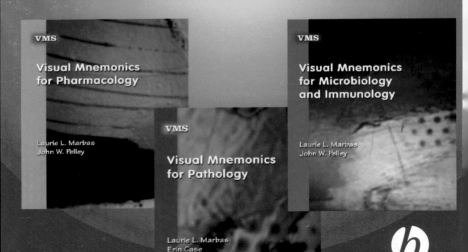